Contents

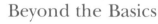

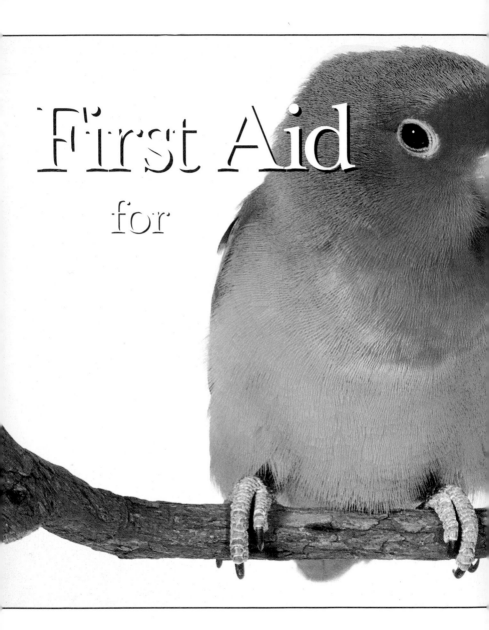

First Aid
for

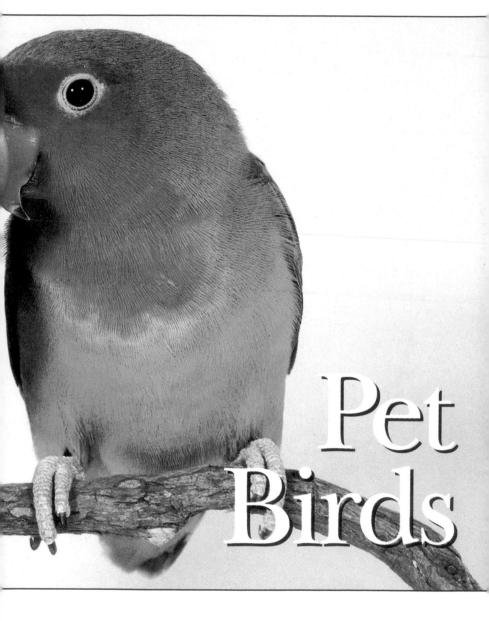

part one

Pet Birds

External Features of a Bird

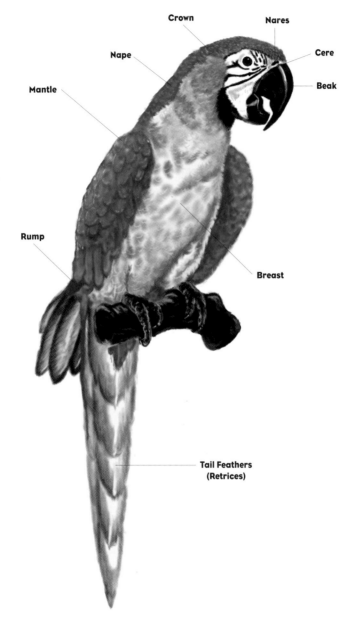

Crown

Nares

Cere

Beak

Nape

Mantle

Rump

Breast

Tail Feathers
(Retrices)

chapter 1

What Is First Aid?

First aid is defined as the initial treatment given to an injured or sick animal while waiting for qualified veterinary treatment. In some cases of minor injury, birds need only to receive first aid at home, while in other cases, first aid is the first step in treating a serious injury or illness. It cannot be viewed as a substitute for qualified avian veterinary care.

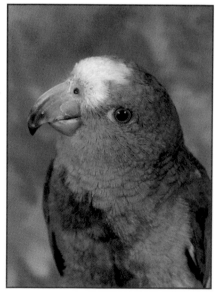

This book is divided into two parts: The first is designed to provide you with first aid information to help you care for your feathered friend when he needs you the most, while the second is meant to help you prevent as many accidents and illnesses as possible.

What Constitutes an Emergency?

A medical emergency is a serious and/or potentially life-threatening injury or disease that requires immediate care. In some instances, such as bleeding, first aid at home may actually be the best first course of action. In addition to any home care, you should contact your avian veterinarian's office immediately in emergency situations for follow-up instructions.

Here are some guidelines from veterinarian Tim Hawcroft on when to call your avian veterinarian:

Call immediately when:

- your bird doesn't stop bleeding
- your bird has blood in droppings or in regurgitated food
- your bird has extensive burns
- your bird has collapsed or can't maintain his balance
- your bird has been poisoned
- your bird has a puncture wound or deep cut
- your bird cannot breathe
- your bird is straining to pass a dropping or an egg

Call the same day when:

- your bird has lost his appetite
- your bird has an eye injury
- your bird has swallowed a foreign object
- your bird has low body temperature
- your bird is mutilating his skin
- your bird has loose droppings
- your bird develops a sudden swelling on his body

Call the next day when:

- your bird is excessively thirsty
- your bird seems to have itchy skin

Bird owners are frequently unsure if a problem is truly an emergency. The best remedy is to follow your instincts and use good common sense. If there's any doubt in your mind regarding the severity of your bird's condition, it's best to treat it as an emergency!

Record Normal Appearance and Behavior

One of the best ways to detect an emergency situation in your pet bird is to know what is considered normal for your bird. Be aware of how much food he eats and how much water he drinks on a regular basis. Know how many times he eliminates in a day and what a normal dropping looks like for your bird. Pay attention to his activity level and his sleeping times.

If your bird is damaging his skin, he should be seen by the veterinarian the same day the condition is noticed.

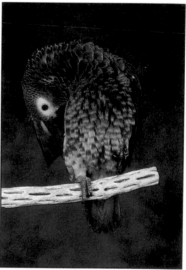

When you are attuned to your bird's normal behavior, you'll notice anything abnormal or unusual right away. In time, you'll even begin to sense when something isn't right about your bird's appearance or behavior, even when the changes are subtle. Listen to that nagging little voice in the back of your head— if something doesn't seem right about your bird, call your avian veterinarian's office for an appointment. Let your avian veterinarian know about any changes in your pet's routine as soon as you notice it so follow-up care, such as a physical examination to rule out injury or illness, can take place promptly.

A Pet Bird First Aid Kit

Before we address the specific techniques, we'd like to suggest that you assemble a bird owner's first aid kit so that you will have some basic supplies on hand before your bird needs them. Here's what to include:

- appropriate-sized towels for catching and holding your bird

- a heating pad, heat lamp or other heat source

- a pad of paper and pencil to make notes about your bird's condition

- address and phone number of your avian veterinarian's office, along with address and phone number of your closest animal emergency hospital

- styptic powder, silver nitrate stick or cornstarch to stop bleeding (use styptic powder and silver nitrate stick on beak and nails only)

- blunt-tipped scissors

- nail clippers and nail file

- needle-nosed pliers (to pull broken blood feathers)

- blunt-end tweezers

- hydrogen peroxide or other disinfectant solution

- eye irrigation solution, such as a saline solution or wetting solution for contact lenses

- basic bandage materials such as gauze squares, masking tape (it doesn't stick to a bird's feathers like adhesive tape) and gauze rolls

- Pedialyte or other energy supplement, such as orange juice or Gatorade

- eye dropper

- syringes to irrigate wounds or feed sick birds

- penlight

- cotton swabs to apply medication and clean wounds

- Betadine soap, which is an anti-infective soap, for foot injuries

- Betadine solution for open wounds (use this under veterinary advice only)

Keep all these supplies in one place, such as a fishing tackle box. This will eliminate having to search for some supplies in emergency situations, and the case can be taken along to bird shows, on trips or left for the bird-sitter if your bird isn't an adventurer.

First Aid Priorities

In an emergency situation, try to keep calm and work in an orderly process. You should first determine whether the injury or illness is life-threatening. If there are multiple injuries, prioritize your efforts according to the severity of each injury.

LIFE-THREATENING INJURIES OR ILLNESSES

Severe bleeding or blood flowing freely from a wound must be attended to immediately. Treat such life-threatening injuries or illnesses by administering first aid without delay and then calling the veterinarian.

NON–LIFE-THREATENING INJURIES OR ILLNESSES

Injuries or illnesses that are causing distress or pain but are not life-threatening, such as fractures, diarrhea or vomiting, should be treated next. You should be preventing the injury or illness from worsening and preparing the bird for transportation to the veterinarian.

MINOR INJURIES OR ILLNESSES

Injuries such as a superficial abrasion or minor cut come last in the order of priorities for treatment. Care for the bird at home if you know how to treat the condition. Take the bird to the veterinarian if the injury or illness does not improve or if the condition worsens.

SIGNS OF ILLNESS

Some signs of illness in pet birds include:

- a fluffed-up appearance
- a loss of appetite
- sleeping all the time
- a change in the appearance or number of droppings
- weight loss
- listlessness
- drooping wings
- lameness
- partially eaten food stuck to the bird's face or food has been regurgitated onto the cage floor
- labored breathing, with or without tail bobbing
- runny eyes or nose
- not talking or singing

If your bird shows any of these signs, please contact your veterinarian's office immediately for further instructions. Your bird should be seen as soon as possible to rule out any illnesses.

Shock

Any emergency, severe insult to the body or excessive handling can result in shock. Common symptoms of shock include a "depressed," weak, "fluffed-up" look and rapid shallow breathing. If a bird in shock is given intensive treatment and/or handling, the bird may collapse and die on the spot. In a life-threatening injury or illness, simultaneously treat the bird for shock and for the injury or illness.

Simply put, shock is the circulatory system's failure to supply adequate blood flow to meet the body's needs.

The treatment of lower priority (non–life-threatening) injuries and illnesses should be delayed if the bird is in shock.

Urgent Care "Don'ts"

- Don't give a bird medications for humans or medications prescribed for another animal unless so directed by your veterinarian.

- Don't give your bird medications that are suggested by a friend, a store employee or a physician who treats humans.

- Don't give a bird alcohol or laxatives.

- Don't apply any oils or ointments to your bird unless your veterinarian tells you to do so.

- Don't bathe a sick bird.

There are a few things to keep in mind when facing a medical emergency with your pet. First, keep as calm as possible because your bird is already excited from being injured. Your bird will sense your stress and you will just exacerbate this distress. Next, stop any bleeding, keep the bird warm and minimize handling him.

After you've stabilized your pet, call your veterinarian's office for further instructions. Tell them, "This is an emergency," and that your bird has had an accident. Describe what happened to your pet as clearly and calmly as you can. Listen carefully to the instructions you are given and follow them.

Although you should not handle an injured or sick bird excessively, you may need to handle your pet in order to take him to the veterinarian's office for follow-up care after you've administered first aid at home.

When handling your pet, make sure to move slowly and talk to him in a calm, reassuring voice. Finally, transport your bird to the vet's office as quickly and safely as you can.

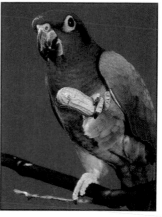

Restraining Your Bird

To make capturing your injured or sick pet bird easier, towel him before you put him in his carrier for the trip to your veterinarian's office. (If you will be transporting the bird in his cage, the toweling step is unnecessary.) Towels make pet birds easier to handle, and they give the birds something to chew on besides an owner's fingers or clothes if the bird is frustrated with the toweling process. In emergency situations, injured or sick birds, even long-time pets, are more prone to bite their owners because

Be aware of your bird's normal activities. Changes can signal illness, and you'll want to take action right away.

they are in pain, don't feel well or are frightened. Having the bird wrapped in a towel in these situations helps an owner protect his or her fingers and transport the pet safely.

Use a towel appropriate to your bird's size. Budgies, canaries and lovebirds can be toweled with washcloths, and kitchen dish towels work well for medium-sized birds. Bath towels are suitable for larger parrots.

How to Towel a Bird

To towel a bird, drape the towel over your hand loosely and reach into your bird's cage. Catch the bird's head with your toweled hand and lift the bird off his perch. As you bring the bird out of his cage, wrap

> **IN AN EMERGENCY**
>
> Bird owners should keep the following tips in mind when facing a medical emergency with their pets:
>
> 1. Keep calm.
> 2. Safely restrain your bird and control bleeding.
> 3. Keep your bird warm and handle him as little as possible.
> 4. Call your avian veterinarian's office for instructions and to alert them that your pet is in need of emergency assistance.
> 5. Safely transport your bird in his cage or carrier to your avian veterinarian's office or animal emergency clinic.

11

An injured bird should be wrapped in a towel to prevent biting and to protect both pet and owner.

the loose ends of the towel around the bird's wings and feet, but don't confine the bird too tightly.

When you've completed the toweling process, your bird should be secure in the towel, but not wrapped so tightly that he is unable to breathe. Keep the towel off your bird's face, and be sure to not constrict the bird's body wall in any way. Birds need to be able to inhale and exhale easily, and they don't have diaphragms as we do to help them breathe, so their body wall must be able to expand and contract for breathing. Your avian veterinarian can give you a demonstration on how to towel a parrot.

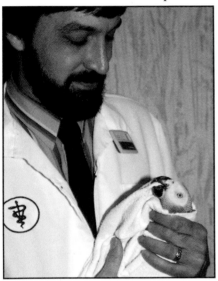

Parrot behavior consultant Mattie Sue Athan reports that parrots show less fear of towels when their owners use towels that are the same color as the parrot. Any neutral, solid-colored towel that doesn't have a lot of loose threads should suffice for toweling a parrot.

When you restrain a bird in a towel, keep the following pointers in mind:

- Work quickly to minimize handling time. Stress and overheating problems will be reduced.
- Plan ahead. Have all tools, equipment and medications ready *prior to restraint.*
- For small birds especially, a net would be helpful to catch the bird if he escapes.
- Towel selection is based on the size of the bird. It will be chewed on, so choose an old one!
- In pet birds, the beak causes injuries. Respect it and protect yourself.
- Birds have very fragile bones. Their legs and wings are most susceptible to injury.
- Don't put any pressure on the bird's chest while holding it. It will interfere with breathing.

- It may help to darken a room just prior to catching birds. The darkness temporarily "freezes" them.

If you are catching small birds, such as canaries or finches, darken the room, then shine a small flashlight in the cage to locate the birds just before you catch them. This technique is not recommended for parrots and larger birds because of their tendency to bite when frightened.

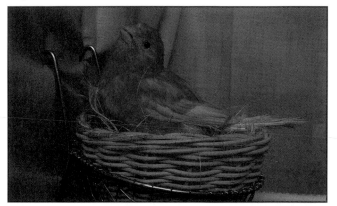

Catching a small bird is easier to do in a darkened room—the sudden lack of light temporarily "freezes" the bird in place.

For larger birds, catch the birds with a towel by letting them out of their cages and gently herding them into the corner of a room that has a hard floor, such as a kitchen or bathroom.

In the case of both small and large birds, you must move decisively to catch them in a towel. Hesitating or having to make a second or third try at catching the bird increases your chances of being bitten. For your safety, you must control your bird's head first (to prevent him from biting you with his beak), and you must release it last.

After you have the bird in the towel, you can restrain him with a three-point hold by placing his head between your thumb and middle fingers, with your index finger across the top of his head, then wrap the rest of the bird's body in the towel to secure his wings and body. Maintain firm pressure on the bird's head, but don't apply too much pressure to the bird's body because the bird needs to breathe freely and the towel keeps his body under control.

Once you've toweled the parrot and removed him from his home, put him in his carrier quickly. Birds left in towels for extended periods of time may become overheated.

Transporting Your Injured or Sick Bird

Call your avian veterinarian's office *before* leaving the house. Explain that you have an emergency and explain what that emergency is so the veterinarian's office can be ready for your arrival. Ask if a veterinarian will be available to see the bird.

By taking this one step, you will save time once your bird has arrived at the veterinarian's office because the staff will have had time to prepare equipment, medication and personnel to treat your bird immediately upon your arrival. By calling ahead, you will also ensure that an avian veterinarian is on hand to treat your bird when you arrive. Finally, you can receive directions to an animal emergency hospital or another hospital that sees birds, which you can drive to directly.

Try to enlist a driver so you can be available to watch your bird and reassure him. If that isn't possible, load your bird into the back seat of your car on the passenger side so you can see him and he can see you during the drive to the veterinarian's office.

If your bird is conscious, provide food within easy reach during transport. Remove water bowls just before leaving home to reduce the chance of spillage. Remove toys and perches from the cage to help protect your bird from further injury on the ride to the veterinarian's office. Cover the cage to reduce stress and provide additional warmth. Do not clean the cage. The as-is environment may help your veterinarian determine the cause of your pet's illness.

Move the bird in his own cage if possible. If that isn't possible, use a cardboard box or pet carrier. Pad the carrier floor with a towel. If you're transporting a small bird, place a hot water bottle under the towel to provide warmth if it's cold outside. Punch ventilation holes in the box if needed. If you aren't taking the bird to the veterinarian's office in his cage, bring along the cage tray liner—this can provide important clues to your veterinarian regarding the cause of your pet's illness.

Whenever you take your pet to the avian veterinarian, you will need to have him restrained in a cage or carrier. At the very least, a cardboard box with a secure lid and some ventilation holes will do, but taking the bird in his own cage is ideal for the veterinarian to be able to analyze the bird and his environment.

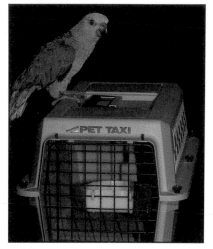

In an emergency, you may be tempted to rush your pet to the veterinary hospital without confining him in his cage. Please take the time to put your pet in a carrier or cage. Your bird could easily fly out of an open car window or be injured severely in the event of an accident if he is not in a secure carrier or cage while traveling in your car.

When it's not possible to transport your bird in his own cage, a pet carrier with a padded floor will suffice.

chapter 2

First Aid
Procedures

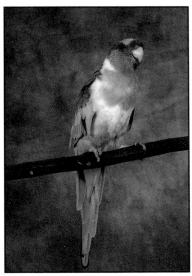

This chapter not only addresses many of the urgent medical situations that bird owners are likely to encounter, but also explains how to prevent them; the reasons they are medical emergencies; signs of illness your bird may exhibit; recommended at-home treatments for the problem; and what course of treatment your avian veterinarian is likely to follow once the bird arrives at the clinic or hospital.

The following information suggests safe and simple guidelines for you to follow when your bird is injured or ill. However, they are not intended to replace veterinary medical care. In medical emergencies that concern your pet bird, always consult your veterinarian first. If his or her advice is contrary to the recommendations we suggest, follow your veterinarian's advice—he or she has the advantage of conducting a hands-on examination of your pet, as well as having the knowledge of your bird's physical condition and her medical history.

The Physical Examination

When you first arrive at the veterinarian's office, let the staff know immediately if your bird is in critical condition. The veterinarian will likely perform a rapid initial exam to determine the extent of the injuries or illness and then begin life-saving treatment that includes fluid and/or oxygen therapy. Once the bird has received this initial treatment, the veterinarian will want to conduct a complete physical exam and to take a history of the bird's health. Be prepared to tell the veterinarian the following information:

- the bird's age and sex (if known)
- how long you've had the bird and how you acquired her
- the type of cage she lives in
- any prior medical problems the bird had
- what the bird has been eating
- what the bird's activity level has been like
- the reason the bird is at the clinic
- what home treatments you've tried before bringing the bird to the clinic
- what signs of illness you have seen in the bird
- what changes in the bird's behavior you've noticed

Note: If you think your bird ingested or inhaled some type of poison, bring the product and its manufacturers' container along.

Shock

Shock is a critical situation that occurs when the cardiovascular system fails to supply adequate blood to the organs of the body. As a result, low blood pressure develops and the cells in the body do not receive adequate amounts of nutrients and oxygen. Shock may follow any serious insult or trauma to the body, including bleeding, severe infection, dehydration, prolonged diarrhea, vomiting or poisoning. If left untreated, shock frequently results in death.

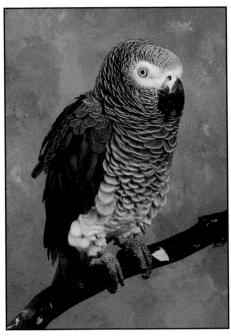

Although this bird's feathers are fluffed, she isn't in shock. "Shocky" birds are weak and act depressed in addition to having fluffed feathers.

Birds that are in shock will appear weak, act depressed, breathe rapidly and have a fluffed-up appearance. If your bird displays these signs, shock should be suspected.

If you believe that your bird is in shock, keep her warm, cover her cage and transport her to your veterinarian's office immediately. Be sure to call your veterinarian's office first. Make sure they are open, that there is a veterinarian on duty and give them time to prepare for the emergency.

Once your bird arrives at the veterinary hospital, your veterinarian will immediately examine the bird, get a brief history and begin treatment. This will include administering fluids to hydrate the bird and oxygen to ease difficult breathing, warming the bird, administering "shock-specific" drugs as needed and closely monitoring the bird.

Once your bird is stable, diagnostic tests will likely be recommended. These can be very important to better assess the extent of the injuries, offer a realistic prognosis and monitor the response to treatment

Loss of Appetite

Birds usually lose their appetite when they are sick or injured. Loss of appetite is not a diagnosis. It is simply the result of a medical problem and serves as an indication that there is a problem with your bird. Remember, healthy birds have healthy appetites!

When a bird suddenly loses her appetite, it's easy for an observant owner to notice. However, when a bird gradually loses her appetite, it may be more difficult to notice, especially if the decrease in food consumption is not a significant quantity.

If you suspect your bird isn't eating as much as she normally does, weigh her at home. Bird owners should make a habit of weighing their pets regularly and keeping this information in a written record. Weight loss can be a good early indicator of a medical problem. Concerns should arise when weight loss approaches 10 percent of the normal weight for your bird. It is essential to purchase a reliable scale that weighs in grams, not ounces. Gram scales are much more accurate at detecting small, but significant, changes in weight.

Birds have rapid metabolic rates and as a result require many calories in relation to their small size to maintain their optimum body weight. Therefore, if small parrots, such as budgies and cockatiels, go for more than twelve hours, and larger parrots go for more than twenty-four hours without food, an emergency situation may be developing.

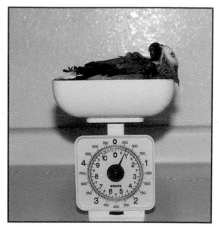

Periodically weigh your bird on a gram scale—a loss of weight may indicate an underlying health problem.

If you notice that your bird eats less food than usual or refuses to eat altogether, try to tempt her with a variety of favorite foods. Warming your bird's food may make eating more appealing. You can also try to feed your bird by hand or with a spoon. If after a short period of time, there is no improvement in appetite, call your veterinarian.

Your veterinarian may need to "force-feed" your bird by gently passing a feeding tube into her crop and instilling a liquid diet that is high in quality and in calories. Once the bird is stabilized with nutrients, fluids and possibly medications, it is important to try to determine the underlying cause of the loss of appetite. After this is done, more specific therapy can be administered. In addition, there are medications that can be used to stimulate your bird's appetite.

Common Diagnostic Tests

Birds cannot communicate with us, and generally hide or cover up signs of disease very well. As a result, veterinarians have to depend not only on a thorough history and complete physical exam, but also on diagnostic tests to uncover the actual cause of the medical problem.

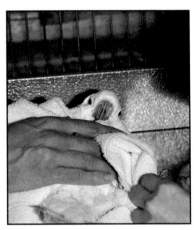

Your avian veterinarian may draw blood from your bird to screen for infection, inflammation, anemia, blood parasites and protein levels.

There are a few commonly performed diagnostic tests that can be especially useful in an emergency situation and will be mentioned throughout this section of the book. Brief descriptions of these valuable and informative tests are included here.

COMPLETE BLOOD COUNT AND DIFFERENTIAL

A complete blood count and differential is an excellent initial screening test for the presence of infection, inflammation, anemia, blood parasites and protein levels. It obtains packed cell volume (also known as PCV or hematocrit), plasma protein concentration, total white blood cell count and includes a blood film examination for the differential white blood cell count, blood cell appearance and a platelet count estimate.

BLOOD CHEMISTRIES

Evaluation of chemical components in the blood provides important information that helps to formulate an accurate diagnosis, prescribe proper therapy and monitor response to therapy. These assays look for imbalances in certain biochemical functions, which when present could point to the possibility of organ dysfunction.

RADIOGRAPHS OR "X-RAYS"

The ability to "see" inside the body is one of the most valuable diagnostic tools available. Bone abnormalities, size and appearance of most internal organs, presence of foreign bodies or soft tissue masses, such as tumors, and much more can be evaluated with radiographs.

BACTERIAL CULTURE/SENSITIVITY AND FUNGI/YEAST CULTURE

Our ability to identify and even prevent many infectious diseases is greatly enhanced by this group of diagnostic tests. A sterile cotton-tipped swab is used to carefully collect a specimen for gram stain and culture from an infected area. These tests used together identify the specific bacteria, fungi or yeast present and their approximate numbers. The bacterial sensitivity portion then identifies which antibiotics would be most effective in treating the infection, if it's bacterial in origin.

General Supportive Care

A commonly used medical term and one that appears throughout this section is "general supportive care." This simply means basic medical care from which most sick birds will benefit, regardless of the illness. This term can apply to care administered both at home and in the veterinary hospital. However, the breadth and scope of general supportive care administered in a hospital setting is much more sophisticated and beneficial for the patient.

At home, general supportive care should include keeping the bird warm, making sure she has easy access to food and water, keeping her quiet and calm and watching the bird for signs of improvement or deterioration in her condition.

In the veterinary hospital, general supportive care could include warmth, oxygen therapy, fluid therapy, "force-feeding" and nebulization therapy (a mist or spray of water that may contain medication). In addition, this care would also include close monitoring by the attending veterinarian and the trained support staff.

Emergencies

The signs that indicate an avian medical emergency, home treatment, follow-up care and prevention of the most common emergencies that can affect pet birds follow.

ANIMAL BITES

Bites can be life-threatening emergencies. Animal bites not only cause the obvious puncture wounds but also the potential for the not-so-obvious serious internal injuries and fractures resulting from the "crush" of the animals jaws. Serious infections can develop from being bitten or from being scratched. Once bacteria gain entry into the body from even a very small puncture wound, they can spread via the bloodstream and develop rapidly into a life-threatening situation.

The first forty-eight hours after an animal bite is a critical time period. Even if your bird appears bright and alert immediately following an attack, within this window of time, serious infection could develop.

Signs

Sometimes bite marks can be seen, but often they are hidden by the feathers. Look for general signs of trauma, which could include blood, matted feathers, lameness, "droopy" wing, unsteadiness on the perch or an unusual increase of feathers in the cage or on the house floor.

Home Treatment

There is really no effective home treatment. Call your veterinarian's office and transport the bird there immediately.

Veterinary Treatment

Your bird will first be checked for stability, and if she appears severely injured and in shock, treatment will begin immediately. On the other hand, if your pet appears stable, a complete physical exam will be given first and this will be followed by appropriate treatment which will invariably include the administration of antibiotics. Diagnostic tests may include radiographs to examine for bone and internal injuries and a blood test.

Prevention

Be careful and use common sense when keeping birds with other pets, especially dogs and cats. If you do have your bird out of her cage when other pets are around, supervise them closely.

BEAK INJURY

A beak injury is an emergency because a bird needs both her upper and lower beak to eat and preen properly. Infections can also set in rather quickly if a beak is fractured or punctured.

Beak injuries often occur after a bird has been attacked by another bird, after the bird flies into a windowpane or a mirror, or if she has a run-in with an operating ceiling fan.

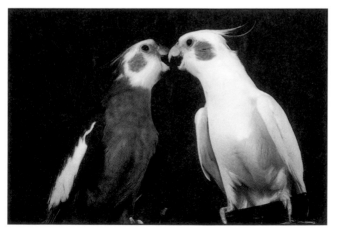

To prevent injury due to aggressive behavior, always closely supervise your pets when they are interacting.

Signs

An injured beak may be cracked, punctured or partially missing. Blood may also be noted coming from the beak or the skin adjacent to the injured area.

23

Home Treatment

Control the bleeding (refer to the section below on bleeding to learn how to do this). Keep the bird calm and quiet. Contact your avian veterinarian's office.

Veterinary Treatment

A complete physical and thorough exam of the beak is necessary before any recommendations can be made. Minor injuries can be cleaned and medicated and you will probably need to follow up at home with antibiotics. More serious injuries could require surgery to repair the damaged beak.

A bird with a beak injury is usually reluctant to eat. This could last for just a few days or for up to a week or even longer. Try offering softer foods, food cut into very small pieces or warmed food. In some instances, some form of "force-feeding" may be required.

Prevention

Prevent your bird from flying, and possible injury, by regularly trimming her wings.

Keep your bird's wings properly trimmed to prevent her from flying into walls or windows. Turn off fans when your bird is out of her cage. Birds have been known to occasionally attack one another, so be careful when birds, especially larger parrots, are kept together. Also be careful when other household pets, especially dogs and cats, come in contact with your pet bird.

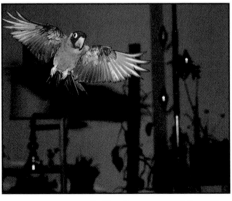

BLEEDING—INTERNAL

Internal bleeding should always be considered life-threatening. This condition could be caused by trauma, a foreign body, cancer, poison, infection or a bleeding disorder (blood fails to clot normally).

Signs

Internal bleeding is evidenced by blood coming from the mouth, nares or vent. Even if the bleeding appears to be intermittent, rather than continuous, or if you notice some dried specks of blood, it should be considered very serious. Blood in the droppings could be seen as fresh "red" blood or the feces could appear black, almost tarlike.

Home Treatment

No home treatment should be attempted. Call your avain veterinarian's office and ask to be seen immediately.

Veterinary Treatment

In order to effectively treat internal bleeding, your veterinarian will need to determine the cause of the bleeding and where in the body it is occurring. This is when a thorough history, complete physical exam and usually diagnostic testing are most important. Once the source has been determined, appropriate treatment will begin immediately. As always, general supportive care will be administered on an as-needed basis. Fluid therapy to hydrate the bird is very important and even blood transfusions are sometimes required.

BLEEDING—EXTERNAL

External bleeding is evidenced by blood seen on the bird's beak, feathers, nails or skin. Owners should be suspicious of any hint of blood on the bird, in her cage, on her playpen, toys or other areas where she has recently been.

IF YOUR BIRD IS BLEEDING

In her book, *The Parrot in Health and Illness*, Bonnie Munro Doane offers the following tips for dealing with birds that are bleeding:

1. Always handle the bird gently and calmly.

2. Always observe the bird for at least one hour after the bleeding has stopped to make sure that it has not restarted.

3. If bleeding has not stopped after a few minutes of treatment, take the bird to the veterinarian immediately.

4. If any signs of listlessness, weakness, paralysis or breathing difficulty are noted, take the bird to the doctor immediately.

5. If bleeding continues, necessitating a trip to the veterinarian, try to have another person drive so that you can continue to apply pressure to the bleeding area.

Home Treatment

The first thing you should do is to stop the bleeding. Try and determine the source of the blood. Read on for more complete instructions.

External bleeding can sometimes be caused by an overgrown beak, as in the case of this cockatiel.

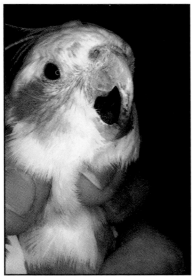

Veterinary Treatment

Your veterinarian may try to stop bleeding through a variety of methods, including cauterization (the sealing of blood vessels with electric current or chemicals), by applying bandages, direct pressure and, if necessary, surgery. A complete exam is essential and this may be followed by a blood test to determine the amount of blood that has been lost. General supportive care, including antibiotics for infection, will be used if needed. Blood transfusions are available but not commonly used.

BLEEDING DUE TO A BROKEN NAIL OR BEAK

If your bird breaks a nail or injures her beak and the bleeding does not stop on its own, catch the bird and apply direct pressure to the injury using a towel or your finger. If a minute or two of direct pressure doesn't work, try applying styptic powder. Be sure to keep the styptic powder out of the bird's mouth.

Observe the bird for at least an hour after bleeding stops. If a piece of nail or beak is cracked or dangling from its base, it will need to be carefully removed. If blood loss is considerable or if your bird seems weak and unsteady, call your veterinarian's office immediately for further instructions.

BLEEDING DUE TO A BROKEN BLOOD FEATHER

In the case of a broken blood feather, you may have to remove the feather shaft from its follicle to stop the bleeding. If you do not do this, the broken feather could continue to bleed, or even become infected.

Follow these steps when treating a broken blood feather. This requires two people—one to restrain the bird and one to remove the feather.

1. Act immediately and restrain the bird.

2. Using firm pressure and sturdy tweezers or needle-nosed pliers, pull the feather out. To do this, grasp the feather as close to the skin as possible. Be gentle and apply smooth, even pressure. If you are removing a broken wing feather, be sure to firmly hold and support the wing as the feather is pulled out. Your assistant will need to very carefully apply equal and opposite traction on the opposite end of the wing as you remove the feather.

   (*Note:* Bird bones are fragile and there is a risk of causing a bone to fracture. Therefore, consider have an avian veterinarian remove the damaged feather.)

3. After the feather is removed, bleeding from the empty follicle may occur. If this happens, apply direct pressure for one or two minutes using a cotton ball or your fingers.

4. Once the bleeding is controlled, observe the bird for at least another hour. The bleeding could recur.

5. Provide supportive care.

6. If blood loss seems excessive or the bird appears weak and listless, *call your veterinarian immediately.* If possible, have another person drive so you can watch the bird closely and help control any bleeding.

BLEEDING DUE TO SKIN WOUNDS

For minor skin wounds that are bleeding, apply direct pressure. If the bleeding doesn't stop with direct pressure, apply a coagulant. If the bleeding stops, observe the bird for several hours. Be aware that birds sometimes will pick at their wounds and, as a result, the bleeding could start again.

If you can't control the bleeding, call your veterinarian and arrange for an office visit. Excessive blood loss may require fluid replacement and, possibly, antibiotic medication to prevent infection. If your bird has a severe wound, surgery may be indicated.

DIFFICULTY BREATHING

Anytime an animal is having difficulty breathing, it certainly must be considered life-threatening. If in respiratory distress, a bird's condition can rapidly deteriorate.

Signs

Wheezing, rapid breathing, open-mouthed breathing and nasal discharge are obvious signs of respiratory distress. Less obvious signs could include tail bobbing (pronounced up and down motion of the tail), frequent stretching of the neck, swelling around the eye, loss of voice and sometimes a "clicking-like" sound when breathing.

Home Treatment

Keep the bird warm, keep the environment calm and relaxed and consider placing a towel over the cage to help reduce your bird's stress level. Also, turning on a vaporizer near the cage for short periods of time or placing your caged bird in a "steamy" bathroom may help ease labored breathing. Call your veterinarian's office and ask to have your bird seen immediately.

Veterinary Treatment

Your veterinarian will first examine your bird and take her medical history. Your bird may be immediately started on oxygen therapy, nebulization and appropriate medications. Once the bird is stabilized, diagnostic tests will probably be recommended to determine the underlying cause of the breathing problem. Specific treatment will then be started.

BURNS

Burns can be very serious and very painful to the bird. Shock and subsequent infection could occur.

Exposure to high temperatures (flame, hot liquids, steam or any hot object), electricity or chemicals can cause burns.

Signs

You should assume that your bird burned herself if you witnessed her directly contact one of the items listed above. In addition, burns should be suspected if an area of the skin has a very inflamed, irritated appearance, or if the feathers are greasy or burnt.

Home Treatment

First, try and determine what type of burn your bird has suffered. Remember, burns can occur from such things as water, hot grease, chemicals or electrical sources. The type of burn determines the treatment that should be followed.

If your bird has been burned by *hot water*, mist the burned area with cool water, or if a leg or foot is burned, try and immerse the burned area in cool water to help relieve the pain. An antibiotic with or without a topical anti-inflammatory medication should be applied. To avoid further damaging the feathers, this medication should be either a water-soluble liquid, spray or powder. Do not apply any oily or greasy substances, including butter, because these substances can damage the bird's feathers.

If the bird has been burned by *hot grease*, lightly coat the burned area with flour or cornstarch to help absorb the grease. (See pages 50 through 51 for more information on how to remove grease from a bird's feathers.)

If the bird has been burned by an *acid*, such as toilet bowl cleaner or drain cleaner, gently flood the burned area with cool water to dilute the chemical, then lightly coat the burned area with a paste of baking soda and water.

If the bird has been burned by an *alkali substance*, such as ammonia or lye, gently flood the burned area with cool water to dilute the chemical, then coat the burned area lightly with vinegar.

If the bird has been burned by an *electrical source*, such as chewing on a power cord, first turn off the power and disconnect the cord. No home treatment is recommended.

In all the above examples, only initial first aid care has been provided. It is critical that your avian veterinarian be consulted for further treatment.

Veterinary Treatment

If your bird is critically burned, she may be in shock and will require immediate and aggressive care. If she is not in shock, a thorough history and physical exam will be performed to determine the type of burn and its severity. Antibiotics are usually given to the bird to prevent infection. In addition to general supportive care, other treatments might include special dressings and bandages. Your bird may need to wear a special collar to prevent her from irritating the wound while it is healing.

Prevention

Prevent your bird from being burned by hot liquids or from a hot stove element by keeping her out of the kitchen when meals are being prepared. Keep the bird away from cleaning supplies to reduce the chances of her receiving a chemical burn. Limit the bird's access to power cords to keep her from receiving an electrical burn, and keep her inside her cage if you have lit candles in the house.

CONCUSSION

A concussion is caused by a blow to the head and could lead to a loss of consciousness. This type of injury frequently occurs if a bird flies into a window or a wall.

Signs

A bird that has a concussion may act depressed, lose her balance, show weakness in her wings or legs, make unusual movements of her eyes or entire head or even lose consciousness.

Home Treatment

No home treatment is recommended for a concussion. Protect the bird from further injury and contact your avian veterinarian immediately.

Veterinary Treatment

Shock, if present, will be treated before the actual concussion. A history and physical exam will be needed to

better assess the extent of the injury. General supportive care and other appropriate medications will be used
as needed. Diagnostic testing may be useful to further
determine the seriousness of the injury.

Prevention

Keep your bird's wings trimmed to prevent her from
being able to fly free in your home. Supervise your pet
when she's out of her cage. Watch young birds carefully because they are more clumsy than adults and are
more likely to hurt themselves.

CONSTRICTED TOE SYNDROME

Constricted toe syndrome is dangerous because it can
cause your bird to lose a toe and potentially develop a
serious infection.

Signs

If your bird has a constricted toe, the toe will look
swollen or inflamed. Constricted toe syndrome is often
seen in young birds and may be related to low brooder
humidity or toe injuries, although the exact cause is
unknown.

Home Treatment

Check to see if the bird has a small piece of thread
wrapped around her toe. If so, attempting to remove it
could damage the area even more. In mild cases, soak-
ing the affected toe in warm water and gentle massage
therapy might help. Topical antibiotics and anti-
inflammatory medications may also soothe the painful
toe. However, these treatments could also give the
injury time to worsen and delay your bird from getting
the veterinary treatment she needs. Contact your avian
veterinarian's office for further instructions.

Veterinary Treatment

After a thorough exam, treatment may include careful
removal of strings or fibers around the toe, removal of
infected tissue, warm-water soaks, massage and appropriate dressings. In the most serious cases, surgery
could be necessary.

CONVULSIONS (SEIZURES)

A convulsion, which is a series of violent and involuntary muscle contractions, indicates that there is a very serious underlying medical problem.

Convulsions are not a diagnosis, rather, they are the result of any number of problems that include head trauma, infection, lead poisoning, some nutritional deficiencies, low blood sugar, low blood calcium, heatstroke, neurological disease and epilepsy (brain malfunction causing recurring seizures).

Signs

In the minutes before a convulsion a bird may appear apprehensive and restless. A convulsion may only affect a single wing or leg or could involve the entire body. Specific signs include uncontrolled shaking, trembling or twitching of the entire body or affected limb. The bird may also lose her balance and fall to the floor or even lose consciousness.

Convulsions usually last only a few seconds, but can last up to a minute or two. The time interval between them can vary. They may occur a few minutes apart, or they may occur days or even months apart. In rare instances, they can seem to continue nonstop.

Home Treatment

There is no effective home treatment for convulsions. The underlying cause must be determined and treated to prevent further episodes. However, during a convulsion protect your bird from further injury by removing objects in her cage, such as perches, toys or food dishes. Cover the cage with a towel if this might help to calm the bird. This is an emergency and your avian veterinarian will want to examine your bird immediately. Be sure to call ahead and make sure a veterinarian is on duty and can see your bird.

Veterinary Treatment

If your bird is actually having a convulsion upon presentation, she needs to be examined immediately.

Medication is available to control convulsions. However, to actually prevent them from recurring, the underlying cause should be determined. Once your bird is stabilized, your veterinarian will probably recommend testing to try and determine their underlying cause. There is specific and very effective treatment for many of the causes of convulsions.

"CROP BURN"

"Crop burns" usually occur in baby birds and can range from causing a little swelling and redness of the crop to a much more severe form, which will cause slow weight gains, prolonged weaning times and crop infections.

Hand-feeding formula that is too hot when fed (more than 105° F) or feeding a bird with incompletely stirred formula that has been heated in a microwave are the most common causes.

Signs
In severe cases, a hole will actually be burned through the crop and overlying skin. Formula will leak from the hole and the surrounding feathers at the base of the neck will be moist and matted. Over time, a scab will usually form over the hole. A foul odor may be noted.

Home Treatment
Minor cases will heal spontaneously and do not require any treatment. Severe cases, such as those causing an obvious hole in the skin, will need to be treated by your veterinarian.

Veterinary Treatment
"Holes" in the crop require surgical closure. Part of the exam will include cleaning the burn site and evaluating the extent of the injury. In addition, drugs such as antibiotics, antifungals or anti-inflammatories will be used.

Prevention
Crop burns can be prevented by paying close attention to the proper temperature of the formula while

heating it, stirring the hand-feeding formula, and by being very careful when heating formula in a microwave. Microwave heating can create "hot spots" within the formula that can easily burn the crop.

DIARRHEA

Diarrhea can cause dehydration and a loss of nutrients.

Diarrhea is actually uncommon in pet birds. Excessive urine is much more common and frequently mistaken for diarrhea. Remember, if the stool is solid and formed, it isn't diarrhea. Increased urine will, however, cause the stool to become wet and slightly loose.

Causes of diarrhea can include diet (sudden change in type of food or spoiled food), intestinal infection, poisoning, ingestion of a foreign object, parasites, generalized diseases, egg laying or egg-binding, overtreatment with antibiotics and stress.

A sudden change in the type of food that you feed your birds can cause diarrhea and/or excessively wet droppings— always introduce new foods slowly and monitor how your birds respond.

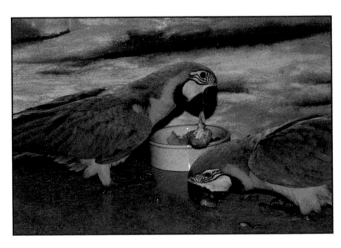

Signs

The signs of diarrhea are loose, watery and unformed stool.

Home Treatment

If your bird has diarrhea, remove any non-food items on which she may be chewing. Feed a bland diet of soft fresh foods, such as pasta, rice, beans and cooked oatmeal. You might consider giving Pepto-Bismol or Kaopectate in the following dosages:

Finches/canaries: 4 drops every 4 hours

"Budgies": 6 drops every 4 hours

Cockatiels: 10 drops every 4 hours

Amazons: 20 drops (1cc) every 4 hours

Cockatoos and macaws: 30 drops (1.5cc) every 4 hours

Remember, any treatment offered at home will delay more specific treatment by your veterinarian. This time delay may be very significant if your bird has a serious health problem.

Veterinary Treatment

Because diarrhea is only the result of a problem and not a diagnosis, veterinarians need to try and determine the underlying cause to more quickly resolve the problem. Therefore, after a thorough history and physical exam, general supportive care will be provided. Diagnostic tests, such as stool analysis and or culture, radiographs and blood tests, may be recommended.

EGG-BINDING

Eggs that remain "bound" inside a hen can lead to very serious medical problems and sometimes even sudden death.

Eggs are usually passed without difficulty and on schedule. However, occasionally such factors as reproductive disorders, excessive egg laying, generalized diseases including infections and nutritional deficiencies or excesses can lead to egg-binding.

Signs

An egg-bound hen will strain to lay eggs unsuccessfully. She may sit on the floor of her cage and may also be panting, depressed, fluffed and lethargic. The eggbound hen may also appear partially paralyzed in one or both legs and may have a swollen abdomen. An egg may or may not be visible from the vent.

Home Treatment

Home care can be attempted; however, if no egg is passed, precious time will be lost. Therefore, please consider contacting your avian veterinarian before trying to treat the problem.

Increase the environmental temperature to 85° to 90° F, increase the humidity. Place her in a "steamy" bathroom. Create a small tent over the cage using plastic sheeting and turn on a vaporizer for about an hour at a time. A wet, warm towel on the cage floor may also help. Regardless of what method you use to raise the humidity, be careful and don't "overcook" your bird!

Provide her with energy supplements in her water source, such as Gatorade, Karo syrup or even a little sugar.

Veterinary Treatment

Treatment, of course, depends on the condition of the bird. After the initial exam and general supportive care, a radiograph may be recommended to not only confirm the diagnosis but also to determine the size, shape and calcium content of the egg. Medication is used to first try and stimulate contractions to aid in pushing the egg out. If medication alone doesn't work, the hen may need to be anesthetized—by relaxing the hen and her muscles, along with a little lubricant, it often allows for the egg to be gently manipulated and removed. If this also fails, other treatments including surgery to remove the retained egg may be necessary.

Prevention

To prevent egg-binding, keep breeding hens healthy and provide them with good diets. If your bird lays eggs, you can try and prevent eggs from being produced by lowering the breeding stimuli in the bird's environment. To do this, remove the nest box from the bird's cage, take away her favorite toys, do not provide her with a mate and limit the bird's exposure to light to between eight and ten hours a day.

Hens with recurring egg-laying problems may be candidates for medications that can prevent eggs from being produced or for surgery to remove the reproductive tract, (i.e., hysterectomy). Discuss these options with your veterinarian.

Eye Injury

All eye problems should be considered potentially serious and could lead to serious infections and even blindness.

Signs

Signs of eye injury include a swollen or closed eye, increased blinking or squinting, rubbing of the eye or discharge from the eye. The surface of the eyeball could lose its normal transparency and appear "cloudy" or "hazy."

Home Treatment

As mentioned, any eye problem should be considered serious. Home treatment will delay proper veterinary care that could mean the difference between saving or losing an eye.

However, home treatment should first include examining the eye carefully for any tiny foreign objects. Obviously, magnification usually helps you see if there is something there. The eye could be rinsed with plain tap water or with over-the-counter eye wash for humans, such as a saline solution or contact lens wetting solution.

No other safe home treatments can be suggested for eye problems. Please consult your avian veterinarian.

Veterinary Treatment

After the history and general exam, the eye will be closely examined. A special eye stain will usually be

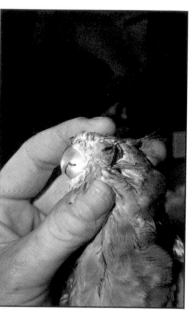

An eye problem should be seen by an avian veterinarian immediately because serious problems, including blindness, could result if the problem is not treated properly.

37

applied to determine if a scratch or abrasion exists on the surface of the eyeball. An opthalmoscope may be used to further examine the inside structures of the eye. Treatment usually consists of eye medications that will need to be instilled into the affected eye several times a day until healed. Surgery is occasionally necessary to repair an injury or to temporarily cover the eye to protect it.

FALLING OFF PERCH

Adult birds are normally surefooted and rarely slip or fall off a perch. If they do, it could be suggestive of a serious underlying problem.

Birds that suddenly become unsteady on their perch may have foot problems, be weak and listless from internal disease or have had a seizure. Regardless of the cause, the problem should be investigated with your avian veterinarian.

A young bird may also have the above problems but may be just learning to perch and is therefore somewhat clumsy.

Signs
The bird suddenly is unsteady or clumsy on her perch.

Home Treatment
Lower perches and remove any objects in the cage that could injure your bird should she fall. Check to make sure all perches are securely attached to the cage walls. Add an energy supplement, such as Gatorade, Karo syrup or simply sugar, to her water source. Call your avian veterinarian and schedule an appointment.

Veterinary Treatment
As mentioned, there are many reasons for birds falling off their perches and just as many treatments. Therefore, the exact cause will need to be investigated. General supportive care will be administered as needed. A thorough history and complete physical exam is essential. Diagnostic tests are generally a very important part

of helping to identify the underlying cause. Specific treatment cannot be started until the diagnosis is known.

Prevention

Keep your birds in optimal health. Pay close attention and be observant for early signs of disease. Remember, young birds naturally tend to be a little clumsy when they are first getting around in their new cage.

FOOT INJURIES

Foot injuries may bleed, cause pain and result in infection. If such an injury is left untreated, birds may chew the affected area and exacerbate the problem.

Foot injuries can result from fractures, toe problems, broken or cracked nails, trauma, frostbite and even from some internal diseases.

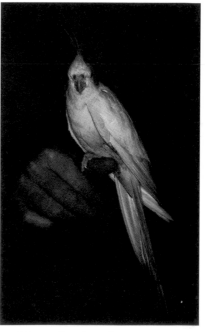

Signs

There may be wounds on the toes of the affected foot. The toes may also be swollen, misshapen or bleeding. Lameness or even non-weight bearing on the affected foot may be apparent.

Home Treatment

Stop any bleeding (see the earlier sections on bleeding). Make your bird comfortable, lower all perches and keep food and water well within easy reach. Contact your avian veterinarian's office for further instructions.

Birds should bear weight evenly on both legs. This cockatiel is lame and is non–weight bearing on her right leg.

Veterinary Treatment

A close and thorough examination of not only the foot, but also the entire leg is very important. A thorough history of the bird's health may help your veterinarian identify the cause. Diagnostic tests, such as a radiograph, to see if a fracture or bone infection is present, or a bacterial/fungal culture may be recommended. Treatment may include topical and systemic medications, bandages for support and protection or surgery.

FRACTURES

Fractures are obviously painful, prevent normal movement and function of the affected limb, but most importantly they are an indication that your pet could have sustained even more serious internal injuries.

Bird bones are brittle and can easily be broken. Pet birds fracture legs more commonly than they fracture wings. Skull and spinal fractures are very serious and are fortunately uncommon.

Fractures are usually caused by accidents. However, poor nutrition and certain diseases can actually weaken bones and make them more susceptible to fractures.

Signs

Fractured leg bone: Non-weight bearing, leg hanging in awkward position. Severe bruising and/or swelling.

Fractured wing bone: Wing hanging lower than other normal wing, inability to move wing, severe bruising and/or swelling.

Fractured skull or spinal cord: Depends on severity and location, but can be as severe as loss of consciousness and/or total paralysis.

Other problems such as arthritis, dislocation, muscle, ligament or tendon injuries and abdominal tumors can present with nearly identical signs.

Home Treatment

Confine the bird to her cage or a small carrier that is padded with a towel. Don't handle your pet unnecessarily. Keep her warm and contact your avian veterinarian.

Veterinary Treatment

Fractures of the legs and wings are usually not life-threatening. However, if your bird is in shock or is very weak, general supportive care will need to be provided first. Once stabilized, and following a complete examination, radiographs will need to be taken. Radiographs can rule out the other problems listed above that can mimic a fracture. In addition, once the severity and location of the fracture is known, the treatment options can be discussed. Bandages and splints can be used to repair many fractures. However, sometimes surgery to internally repair the broken bone is necessary. With proper care, fractures require about four weeks to heal.

FROSTBITE (HYPOTHERMIA)

Frostbite is an emergency because, in a moderate case, the bird's toes could be lost, or, in a severe case, the bird could die.

Signs

The frostbitten area will be very painful, cold and hard to the touch. After several days the affected area may become very hard, dry and dark black in color.

Home Treatment

Place the bird in a warm environment (85° to 90° F). Warm up the damaged tissue very gradually in a warm circulating water bath. Food and water should be easily accessible to the bird. Your avian veterinarian will want to examine the bird.

Veterinary Treatment

Your avian veterinarian will warm the bird gradually by placing her in an incubator and administering warm intravenous fluids. Your bird will also receive a physical examination and supportive care. If, after several days, the affected area does not appear to be healing well, surgery may be necessary.

Prevention

Keep birds indoors during extremely cold weather. Most pet birds can tolerate outdoor temperatures that dip down to 30° F. Cold temperatures combined with dampness and/or wind will create an ideal environ-ment for frostbite to develop. Birds housed outdoors in cold weather should not be kept on metal perches.

HEATSTROKE (HYPERTHERMIA)

Overheated birds can go into shock quickly. Per-manent brain damage or even death can result.

Signs

An environment that is very warm and a bird that is panting, holding her wings down and away from her body. The bird will also be extremely weak and could go into shock or a coma. Young, old or overweight birds are more sus-ceptible to heatstroke than other birds.

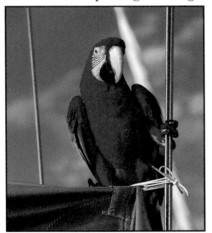

Protect your bird from heatstroke by providing her with shade, cool water and fresh fruit.

Home Treatment

First, remove the bird from her hot environment and place her in a cool area. Start to reduce her body temperature by placing her in an air-conditioned room, in front of a fan, or spraying her with cool water from a misting bottle. Make sure the feathers are wet to the skin. Offer the bird cool water to drink if she is able, or begin to give her a few drops of cool water by mouth. Contact your avian veterinar-ian's office for further instructions.

Veterinary Treatment

In addition to general supportive care, the patient will be placed in a cool, well-oxygenated and moist envi-ronment. Dehydration can be treated by administering fluids. The bird should be closely monitored for at least twenty-four hours.

Prevention

You can reduce your bird's chances of suffering heat-stroke by keeping her out of direct sun, providing her with ample supplies of clean, fresh water and not keeping her in a car on a hot day. Interior temperatures in a car can rise quickly during hot weather, which can cause serious problems for all pets.

INFECTIONS (BACTERIAL, FUNGAL AND VIRAL)

Infections can quickly cause several potentially serious and life-threatening problems.

Signs

Depending on the location of the infection within the body, birds can display any and all general signs of a sick bird. Appetite loss and weakness generally accompany most infections.

Home Treatment

No home treatment is recommended. Call your avian veterinarian for an appointment.

Veterinary Treatment

General supportive care will be provided as needed. Antibiotics, antifungals and sometimes antiviral drugs are available to fight the infection. A bacterial or fungal culture and sensitivity can be very beneficial in determining the best medications to use. Blood tests may also be useful to diagnose an infection and monitor the response to treatment.

INGESTED FOREIGN OBJECT

Ingested foreign objects can cause obstructions, irritate and inflame the lining of the gut and frequently cause other life-threatening problems.

Signs

There are no signs that are distinctively characteristic for a bird that has ingested a foreign object. The bird may regurgitate, have diarrhea or bloody droppings. However, many other problems will cause these same signs.

You should be suspicious that your bird may have ingested a foreign object if she displays any signs *and* was seen playing with a small item, such as the back of an earring or a piece of a toy, that suddenly cannot be found.

Home Treatment
No home treatment is recommended. Contact your avian veterinarian's office.

Veterinary Treatment
In addition to a thorough history and physical exam, radiographs are essential. Radiographs can frequently identify or at least suggest if a foreign object is present in the digestive tract. However, some ingested foreign objects cannot be seen on standard radiographs and special studies using a safe "dye" may be recommended. Some foreign objects may safely pass through the digestive tract, while others may need to be surgically removed.

Prevention
Birds love to chew and gnaw with their beaks. Avoid toys and objects that can be taken apart, broken or chipped. Larger birds need stronger, heavier toys and other objects with which to play.

INHALED FOREIGN OBJECT
Inhaled foreign objects can obstruct major breathing airways. As a result, movement of air through the respiratory tract can be partially or completely blocked.

Signs
If a foreign object gets lodged in the nares or sinuses, signs may only include open-mouth breathing, panting and tiring easily. Look carefully in the nares because a foreign object may be visible. If on the other hand, a small morsel of food or other small object is aspirated into the trachea (i.e., "windpipe"), very serious breathing problems will immediately become apparent.

Home Treatment

No home treatment is recommended. Call your avian veterinarian and tell them your bird's symptoms. You will most likely be seen immediately.

Veterinary Treatment

Your veterinarian will first need to perform an exam. The bird may be placed in an oxygenated cage and given drugs to aid in breathing. If a foreign object is visible, it may be easily and carefully removed. If an object is in the trachea, and breathing is severely compromised, a special breathing tube placed into the lower part of the body cavity can help to significantly improve breathing. Foreign objects in the trachea can, in many instances, be successfully removed.

JOINT SWELLING

Joint swelling can suggest an infection, arthritis, trauma or a dislocation (a displacement of bone out of the joint it helps to form).

Signs

The bird's affected joints are painful, swollen and stiff. If joints in the leg are swollen, the bird will be lame.

Home Treatment

Keep the bird quiet and comfortable and call your avian veterinarian for further instructions. No home treatment is recommended for joint swelling.

Veterinary Treatment

The bird's history and physical exam is very important. Diagnostic tests may be recommended to determine the reason for the joint swelling. To do this, radiographs, joint aspiration (to analyze fluid found in the joint) and blood tests may be needed. Treatment will be prescribed based on the underlying cause.

LEAD AND ZINC POISONING (METAL POISONING)

Lead and zinc poisoning cause serious life-threatening problems in pet birds. These two ingested poisons are grouped together because their sources, signs and treatment are very similar. Lead and zinc are the most common sources of poisoning in pet birds.

Signs

A bird with lead or zinc poisoning generally shows signs involving the digestive and neurological systems. Digestive signs may include vomiting, regurgitation and abnormal droppings that include yellow or green urates and sometimes even blood. Neurological signs may include convulsions, paralysis, twitching, abnormal head movements and blindness. Depression, weakness and appetite loss are also common.

Home Treatment

There is absolutely no recommended home treatment. Lead or zinc poisoning requires early and aggressive veterinary treatment. Make an appointment to see your avian veterinarian immediately.

Veterinary Treatment

Diagnosis may be challenging because pet bird owners often deny any possibility of metal ingestion. History and physical exam are essential but they alone cannot diagnose this problem. Radiographs are very helpful in establishing an early diagnosis because metal particles are often, but not always, seen in the digestive tract. Blood tests to assay for lead and zinc are available but may take a few days to get the results. Because an antidote is available and is very effective, sometimes a dramatic response to treatment will help make a diagnosis. Treatment is aimed at stabilizing the patient, removing the source of the metal from the environment and removing the metal from the body tissues using intestinal lubricants and bulking agents in conjunction with the specific antidote. In addition, antibiotics are given to control the possibility of infection and, as always, general supportive care as needed. Duration of treatment varies and may require several days, weeks and sometimes months to complete.

Lead poisoning can be prevented by removing common sources of lead from your bird's environment. See the "Preventing Lead Poisoning" sidebar for specific items to keep out of your bird's reach. "Lead" pencils won't cause lead poisoning; they're actually graphite.

Zinc poisoning is often caused by birds ingesting pieces of galvanized metal, which are commonly used for outdoor wire cages. Birds can also encounter zinc in washers, nuts, snap fasteners and pennies (pennies minted since 1982 are 97.5 percent zinc).

Outdoor bird cages are often constructed with galvanized wire. These should be avoided; however, there are often no other acceptable substitutes. If your bird or birds are housed in a galvanized wire cage and you cannot replace it, then wash down the cage wires with a solution of vinegar and water, scrub the cage thoroughly with a wire brush to loosen any stray bits of the galvanized wire. Rinse the cage thoroughly with water and allow it to dry before putting it to use. Newly galvanized wire poses a greater poisoning threat than older more "seasoned" wire. Talk to your avian veterinarian for further suggestions on the prevention and control of metal poisoning.

LEG BAND PROBLEMS

If a banded leg gets injured and becomes swollen, a leg band could cause additional

---

PREVENTING LEAD POISONING

Lead poisoning can usually be prevented by keeping birds away from common sources of lead in the environment. These include:

antiques

bases of light bulbs

batteries

bird toys with weights

bullets and buckshot

costume jewelry

curtain weights

dolomite

fishing weights

foil from wine and champagne bottle seals

hardware cloth

lead-framed doors and windows

mirror backing

old paint

old plaster

putty

sheet rock

solder

stained glass ornaments, lampshades and other items

unglazed ceramics

zippers (some types)

damage because a tight band can interfere with normal blood flow in the leg. Leg bands can also get caught on various items in a pet bird's environment and if this happens, the leg would become susceptible to injury.

Signs

Your bird's leg may be swollen or puffy around the leg band, or the band may not be "floating" freely on the bird's leg. Normally, leg bands should fit loosely around a bird's leg.

Home Treatment

If the bird's leg band becomes caught on a toy, her cage or something else, do your best to carefully and

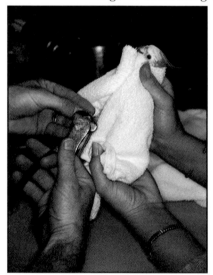

gently undo the entanglement and free the bird. If necessary, carefully use wire cutters to cut wire, or try to take apart whatever the leg band is caught on. Wrap the bird's leg if it is bleeding.

Do not attempt to remove the leg band. Removing leg bands is a very delicate procedure and should only be performed by an experienced person, preferably an avian veterinarian.

Leg band removal is a delicate procedure that should only be attempted by an avian veterinarian.

Veterinary Treatment

If your bird's leg is severely swollen and the band is now snug around the leg, your veterinarian will remove the band. This may require anesthetizing your pet to ensure her safety. Bandaging and supportive care may also be required. If the leg is obviously injured, a radiograph may be recommended to rule out any bone injury.

Prevention

Leg bands are either open or closed. Open leg bands have a small gap in their circle. At one time, these bands were commonly placed on adult birds during the quarantine process of legal importation into this country. However, open bands are no longer used due to a 1992 law that prohibits the importation of birds.

Closed leg bands form a continuous ring and denote a domestically bred bird. These bands are placed on baby birds and, as the bird grows, the band will no longer be able to slip off the leg. The numbers, letters or designs engraved on the band are in code. They usually identify the breeder and the birth date of the bird.

If your bird is an imported bird that has an open leg band, ask your veterinarian to remove the band to protect your pet from injury. If your bird is a domestically bred parrot with a closed leg band, discuss the possibility of removing it with your veterinarian. Some veterinarians recommend leaving closed bands on birds because they can help trace a bird's genealogy. However, if your pet is highly active, removing the band may be in its best interest.

"NIGHT FRIGHTS," "COCKATIEL THRASHING SYNDROME" OR "EARTHQUAKE SYNDROME"

A bird that experiences thrashing episodes will be startled from sleep by loud noises or vibrations that cause her to awaken suddenly and try to take flight. During one of these thrashing episodes, a bird will become highly stressed and could injure herself.

Signs

In the case of caged pet birds, the "thrasher" may injure her wing tips, feet, chest or abdomen on toys or cage bars when she tries to flee from the perceived danger. Cockatiels, particularly lutinos, seem prone to this behavior.

Home Treatment

Assess the bird for bruises, cuts, broken feathers or other injuries. Calm and comfort the bird as best you can. Call your avian veterinarian's office for a checkup.

49

Veterinary Treatment

Your avian veterinarian will perform a physical examination to determine the extent of the injuries. The bird may require treatment for shock or simply for minor injuries.

Prevention

Bird owners can help protect their pets from harm by installing a small night-light near the bird's cage to help the bird see where she is during a thrashing episode, by placing an air cleaner in the bird's room to provide "white noise" that will drown out some potentially frightening background noises, or by placing the bird in a small sleeping cage that is free of toys and other items that could harm a frightened bird.

OILED FEATHERS

Oiled feathers are an emergency because they cause the bird to lose her ability to regulate her body temperature. If a bird falls into oil, she can also suffer from breathing problems, eye problems and poisoning if she swallows any oil.

Signs

Oily, greasy or slick feathers are signs of oiled feathers.

Home Treatment

Contact your avian veterinarian's office for immediate assistance. Cleaning an oil-soaked bird requires multiple steps and for maximum safety should be done by experienced and knowledgeable individuals.

However, if you cannot get your bird to an avian veterinarian immediately, try the following method for removing oil from a bird's feathers:

1. Dust oiled feathers with cornstarch or flour, which helps soak up excess oil. Keep the powder away from the bird's eyes and nose. A suggested method is to place some cornstarch or flour in a small pillowcase or bag, then place the bird inside the bag with her head exposed. Hold the bag around the

bird's neck and gently shake the bag to dust the feathers. Allow the powder to stay on for about thirty minutes. Brush off excess.

2. Wrap the bird in a towel, which reduces heat loss and prevents the bird from ingesting the oil.

3. Remove oil from the bird's nostrils, mouth and around her eyes with a moistened cotton swab.

4. Fill a sink with warm water and add a very small amount of dishwashing soap. Protect the bird's eyes and immerse the bird in the water. Wet all affected feathers by handling them gently and following their natural contour. Dip the bird slowly in and out of the water for one to two minutes. Rinse the feathers well with fresh warm water. Immerse the bird in the soapy water and rinse again as needed.

5. Blot the feathers dry with towels. Do not rub the feathers. A hair dryer set on low is also very useful for drying off the bird.

6. Wrap the bird loosely in a towel and place her in a warm cage, aquarium or box. Increase the environmental temperature to 85° to 90° F for a short time until the bird is dry. Avoid exposing the bird to drafts.

7. Provide general supportive care.

8. If oiling is severe, do not try to remove it all at once. The above steps may need to be repeated over several hours or perhaps even days.

9. Observe the bird closely over the next several hours. Shock and dehydration could develop and are serious concerns.

10. Call your avian veterinarian.

Veterinary Treatment

Your avian veterinarian will perform a physical examination. If the bird is unstable, in shock, dehydrated and/or chilled, these problems will need to be treated first. Once stable, the oiled feathers will be cleaned. Hospitalization and close monitoring may also be part of the treatment for the first twenty-four to forty-eight hours.

Prevention

Limit your bird's access to sources of oil, especially in the kitchen and garage areas.

POISONING

Some poisons can kill a bird quickly. Others can cause clinical signs ranging from a mild digestive tract upset to a violent illness.

Signs

A poisoned bird may suddenly regurgitate, develop diarrhea, bloody droppings, redness or burns around her mouth, go into convulsions, become paralyzed, go into shock or any number of other abnormalities.

NATIONAL ANIMAL POISON CONTROL CENTER (NAPCC)

If your bird is poisoned and you are unable to reach your avian veterinarian's office, you should call the National Animal Poison Control Center (NAPCC) at the University of Illinois, Champaign/Urbana. Phones are answered twenty-four hours a day, and each call is handled by a veterinarian who is specially trained in animal poisoning.

You will need to have a credit card handy before calling because there is a charge for this service, but it could mean the difference between life and death for your bird. The NAPCC's numbers are 800/548-2423 (billed as a flat fee) or 900/680-0000 (billed on a per-minute basis).

Home Treatment

First, try to determine what may have poisoned your pet. Birds can be poisoned by inhaling fumes, by ingesting a poisonous plant or chemical, or by coming in contact with a poison on their skin.

Place the poison out of your pet's and family's reach. Flush the bird's eyes or skin with water if the bird was exposed to the poison in these areas. If the bird is overcome by fumes, open all windows in the room or remove the bird from the room and into fresh air as soon as possible.

Call your avian veterinarian and ask to be seen immediately. Be sure to bring the poison and its original container with you to the veterinarian's office.

Veterinary Treatment

Stabilizing the bird is most important, especially if she is in shock, convulsing or having breathing problems. A complete physical and general supportive care will be given. If an antidote to the poison is available, it will be administered. If ingested, medication can be given to reduce the absorption of the poison into the blood-stream.

Prevention

You can help prevent poisoning in your bird by following these steps:

- Make sure food and water is always fresh.

- Wash all fruits and vegetables before serving them to your bird.

- Keep potentially poisonous household products out of your bird's reach.

- Do not let your bird fly free in the kitchen or bath-room.

- Do not use products with strong fumes, such as cleaning products, around your bird.

- Do not use fungicides, herbicides, insecticides or rodenticides around your bird without consulting your avian veterinarian.

- Do not let your bird near your houseplants.

- Do not leave cigarettes or other tobacco products where your bird can reach them. Ideally, do not smoke around your bird, either.

- Do not use nonstick cookware because overheated nonstick items can emit potentially fatal fumes for your bird.

- Immediately consult your avian veterinarian if you suspect any potential poisoning problems in your pet.

REGURGITATION

Regurgitation, especially in young birds, can indicate a serious health problem. Regurgitation can result from crop infections or blockages, poisoning, thyroid enlargement, infections of the lower digestive tract and other generalized diseases.

In adult birds, regurgitation can also be a normal sign of affection that birds show to a favorite toy or person. In some instances, it can be challenging to determine if the regurgitation is a sign of illness or simply a unique way of showing affection.

Signs

A bird regurgitates undigested food from her crop. The bird may have food stuck to her beak, facial feathers or the top of her head. The feathers on the head may also be sticking together.

Home Treatment

It is difficult to make general recommendations for home treatment because there are many different causes for regurgitation in a sick bird.

In young birds, absolutely no home treatment is recommended. Conditions causing regurgitation can be life-threatening. Call your avian veterinarian immediately for an appointment.

In adult birds, try removing toys or mirrors from the cage if those seem to be stimulating the bird to regurgitate.

Although not particularly effective for this problem, Kaopectate or Pepto-Bismol could be given with a plastic medicine dropper to help soothe an inflamed lining of the digestive tract. (See page 35 for recommended dosages.)

Call your avian veterinarian's office for an appointment if your adult bird doesn't improve in twenty-four hours. Remember, home treatment also delays your pet from receiving more specialized veterinary care.

Veterinary Treatment

Your veterinarian will need a history of when the regurgitation began, how often your bird regurgitates and what stimulates her to regurgitate (if that can be determined). A physical examination and diagnostic tests will likely be recommended to determine the cause of the regurgitation. These may include radiographs, microscopic analysis of the contents of the crop and blood tests.

SELF-MUTILATION

Feathers, skin and toes can be severely damaged by a bird that is picking and gnawing at herself.

Signs

Self-mutilation can be difficult to distinguish from other causes of trauma unless a bird is actually seen picking and chewing at herself.

Home Treatment

Control the bleeding, if any (see the section on bleeding for instructions). Schedule an appointment with your avian veterinarian.

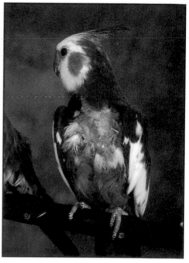

Veterinary Treatment

A history and complete physical exam is most important. Diagnostic tests may be recommended to help differentiate between a medical and behavioral cause for the self-mutilation.

No matter the cause, a restraint collar, bandages or medication should be used to prevent the bird from further injuring herself. There are some very effective behavior-modifying drugs that can help control this obsessive-compulsive behavior.

Self-mutilation, such as feather picking, is usually caused by an underlying behavioral or medical problem.

Antibiotics and anti-inflammatory drugs may also be needed. Once this behavior gets started, even after being cured, it can recur months and sometimes years later.

SLOW CROP EMPTYING

Slow crop emptying indicates that there is a lack of nutrients and energy being supplied to the body. This is a

55

problem most frequently encountered in young birds or very seriously ill adult birds. Some of the problems that can cause a delayed emptying of the crop are bacterial, fungal or viral infections, some poisons, impactions (food or foreign body), enlarged thyroid gland, lower digestive tract diseases and other serious illness. Improperly prepared formula in young preweaned birds can also cause this problem.

Signs

In young birds, a large pendulous crop that fails to empty after several hours suggests a problem. Adult birds have a much smaller crop, even when full, relative to their larger size.

Home Treatment

No home treatment is recommended. Call your avian veterinarian for an appointment.

Veterinary Treatment

The crop is located at the base of the neck. If it is squeezed when full, there is a risk of food being forced back up into the mouth and aspirated into the respiratory tract. Therefore, it is highly recommended that only a veterinarian perform this part of the exam.

After the history and examination, the crop will likely be emptied, lavaged (irrigated or washed out) and its contents microscopically analyzed. Radiographs might also be suggested to rule out foreign objects or obstructions. General supportive care will be provided as needed. Antibiotics and/or antifungal medications are frequently used to regulate the problem. Occasionally, surgery is necessary to remove a foreign object or an obstruction.

TISSUE PROTRUDING FROM THE BIRD'S VENT

There should *never* be anything protruding from a bird's vent.

A protrusion from the vent might be the bird's lower intestines, uterus or cloaca. It could also be a tumor or foreign object. To complicate matters, birds may pick on the protruding tissue and can rapidly make the condition critical.

Signs

If you see anything protruding from your bird's vent, there is a problem. Exposed tissues could appear red, brown or black in color. The bird may also have a bloody beak from picking at the tissue.

Droppings should not be "stuck" or "pasted" around the vent. An egg may be seen protruding, and if it does not get pushed out in a very short time, your bird could be in trouble. See the section on egg-binding on pages 35 through 37.

Home Treatment

No home treatment is recommended. Contact your avian veterinarian's office for immediate care.

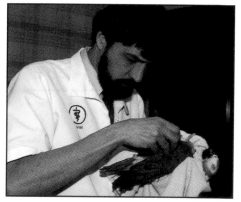

Veterinary Treatment

Your veterinarian will perform a physical examination to confirm the prolapse's severity and likely cause. If it is exposed tissue that recently prolapsed and is still moist and healthy, the tissue may be reduced (gently pushed back inside) with a little lubrication and minor surgery performed to keep it in. Tumors may need to be surgically removed, cauterized (heated or application of a caustic substance) or even frozen. A biopsy should be collected to determine the exact type of tumor and its most effective treatment.

In an emergency situation, your avian veterinarian may want to perform an examination and begin initial treatment to stabilize your bird prior to speaking with you.

In selective cases, major surgery may be required to permanently keep the protruding tissue inside the body.

What to Expect at the Veterinary Hospital

Rushing your bird to your avian veterinarian's office in an emergency situation is a frightening, stressful thing to go through. Try not to take out your feelings on the veterinarian or the staff members. As caring animal lovers, they want to see your pet go home healthy as much as you do.

Keep in mind that your veterinarian may not be able to answer questions or talk with you for an extended period of time when you bring your bird in because he or she may need to begin what could be life-saving treatment on your pet. A staff member may act as a messenger between the veterinarian and you.

In cases of minor emergencies, such as an inhaled seed in the bird's nares, you can wait while the veterinarian treats your bird and take her home with you within the hour. In other cases, where surgery or other treatment is required, it may be best to go home and wait for the veterinarian to call you when your pet is stable.

chapter 3

Home Care
for Recuperating
Birds

Avian emergencies frequently require follow-up care, either in the veterinary hospital or at home. Severely ill birds, such as those needing special care for surgery, shock, seizures, poisoning or severe breathing difficulties, will need to be cared for in the hospital. Other birds may need to be taken to the hospital for daily treatments. However, many birds can receive follow-up care at home, which provides them with a familiar environment in which to recuperate and reduces the cost of follow-up care for owners. You and your veteri-

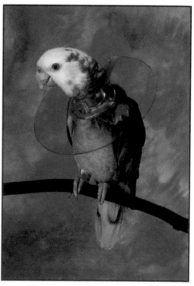

narian can work together to determine when your bird needs hospitalization and when he can recover at home.

Your Recovering Bird's Needs

Sick birds have a few special requirements during their recovery period. They need supplemental heat, food and water, rest and relaxation and observant owners. You may also need to medicate your bird.

SUPPLEMENTAL HEAT

To provide additional heat for a sick bird, you can place a heating pad below the cage or alongside it if the cage is small. Cover the top of the cage and three sides of it to prevent heat loss. Make sure to keep the bird from chewing on the pad.

If your bird lives in a large cage, you can tent it in an electric blanket set on low. Make sure that your bird doesn't chew on the blanket.

You can make a home hospital cage by setting a small aquarium with a screen- or towel-covered roof on a heating pad. If the aquarium floor becomes too warm, check the setting on the heating pad. You can also line the floor with newspaper.

Another way to provide additional heat is to put a red/amber infrared 250-watt heat lamp with a porcelain socket and clamp set-up 2 to 4 feet away from your bird's cage.

In order to monitor temperature properly, you will need to place a thermometer near the floor of the cage you are trying to heat. As in the case of heating pads and electric blankets, keep your bird from chewing on the thermometer. If you are heating a cage, you can hang the thermometer on the outside of the cage near the floor, while wall-mounting aquarium thermometers can be mounted on the outside of the enclosure.

Focus the heat on one side of the cage so your bird can move toward it if he is cold and away from it if he becomes too warm. If your bird is too cold, he will huddle with his feathers fluffed, while he will hold his wings away from his body and pant if he becomes too warm.

NUTRITION

In order to give your bird the best chance at recovery, he must be encouraged to eat and drink water while he is ill. Unfortunately, this is often a difficult task because sick birds usually lose their appetites. Owners can improve their birds' chances at eating by following a few simple steps.

Keeping a recovering parrot full of food is one of a bird owner's primary concerns. You can offer favorite treats by hand to ensure that your pet is eating. You may try holding your bird with one hand and his food bowl in the other. Allow him to choose whatever he wants to eat.

Finally, you will need to weigh your bird daily to see if your efforts at stimulating his appetite are paying off. A gram scale is a more accurate method of weighing your pet bird than a scale that weighs in ounces. Weight loss of more than 10 percent may require that your bird be force-fed with a tube. This may mean that he will have to be hospitalized.

To get your bird to drink enough water while he is ill, you can add fruit juice, Gatorade or Pedialyte (an infant fluid and electrolyte replacement solution that is available at most drugstores). You can use these fluids at full strength or you can dilute them with water. You can also add fruits to your bird's diet if he is eating, or you can moisten cereal or add warm soup to the diet.

If your bird is not drinking enough water, you may have to use an eye dropper or syringe to give the bird small amounts of water by mouth. Recommended amounts of fluid to give at a single sitting are 4 to 5 drops for canaries and finches, 6 to 10 drops for budgies, $\frac{1}{4}$ teaspoon for cockatiels, 1 to 3 teaspoons for medium-sized parrots such as Amazons, and $1\frac{1}{2}$ to 3 tablespoons to large parrots such as cockatoos and macaws. If your bird won't take the full amount at a single sitting, divide up the number of drops and offer some every fifteen to twenty minutes. You should offer the full amount several times a day to ensure your bird has enough fluids in his system.

REST AND RELAXATION

As far as rest and relaxation are concerned, a bird that is relaxed has more energy to get well than one that is under stress. Keep your recuperating bird in a dimly lit, quiet room. Provide him with twelve hours of darkness daily to encourage the bird to sleep and twelve hours of light to encourage him to eat. Do not handle a sick bird unnecessarily, and keep children and other pets away from the recovering bird.

MEDICATION

If your bird has been seen by an avian veterinarian, it is likely that some type of medication has been prescribed to help him recuperate more quickly.

Make sure you understand all the instructions you receive from your veterinarian or animal health technician for medicating your pet, including the amount to be given, number of times the medication is administered daily and how many days the total course of treatment will run, before you leave the veterinary hospital.

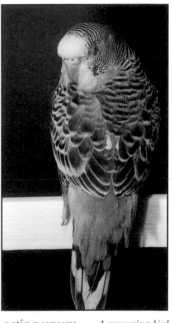

If you forget part of the instructions or if something is unclear once you get home, don't hesitate to call the veterinarian with follow-up questions. If your bird seems to be having a reaction to the medication (regurgitating, shaking or acting unusually), let your veterinarian's office know immediately. A different type of medication may need to be prescribed, and your pet will need to have such reactions noted in his chart.

A recovering bird should be given a calm and stress-free environment in which to rest.

Methods of Medicating Your Bird

The most common methods of administering medications to birds are divided into two categories—systemic and topical. Systemic medications are injected or given orally.

ORAL MEDICATION

It is difficult to orally medicate birds that are small, easy to handle or underweight, but you can successfully medicate any bird. The medication is usually given with a plastic syringe (needle removed) placed in the left side of the bird's mouth and pointed toward the right side of his throat. Give the medication a few drops at a time to minimize the chance of the bird aspirating the medication.

QUESTIONS TO ASK BEFORE MEDICATING YOUR BIRD

- If the bird is to receive the medicine twice a day, do you need to wait twelve hours between doses?

- Is the medicine more effective if the bird has an empty stomach, a full stomach or can the medicine be given regardless of when the bird has last eaten?

- Does the medication need to be refrigerated?

- If the medicine is to be injected, do you have the right number of syringes? How does the veterinary hospital want you to dispose of these syringes after you've used them? Can the staff mark the syringes for you so you can easily determine the correct dosage for your pet?

In most cases, you'll need to safely restrain your bird before administering the medication. To do this, you will need two people: one to hold the bird and one to give the medication. The person holding the bird will need to towel the bird and hold him securely in a three-point hold. (Remember to allow the bird's chest to rise and fall without any pressure or restraint on him.) After the bird is under control, the person giving the medication can administer it quickly with a minimum risk of injury to either bird or people.

You can also medicate a bird orally by giving him medicated feed (such as tetracycline-impregnated pellets), or by putting medication in his food or his water. However, medications added to a bird's water supply are often less effective because sick birds frequently do not drink; moreover, the medicated water may have an unusual taste that does not appeal to the bird.

INJECTABLE MEDICATION

Some avian veterinarians consider this the most effective method of medicating birds. Injection sites are into a vein, beneath the skin or into a muscle. Bird owners are usually asked to inject their birds intramuscularly, i.e., into the bird's chest muscle. This is the area of the bird's body that has the greatest muscle mass, and it is therefore a good injection site.

Pet owners must be thoroughly instructed by a veterinarian on the technique of giving injections before proceeding with medicating their birds at home. Owners may be uncomfortable at first, but will soon find that giving injections is very easy and much less stressful on the bird than giving oral medications.

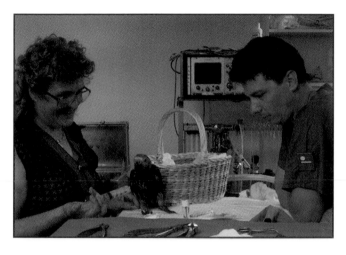

With proper instructions from a veterinarian, bird owners can learn to safely and confidently administer their pet's medication.

Effective restraint is the key to injecting your pet bird safely. Have someone towel your bird and hold him so that you can administer the injection. Insert the syringe at about a 45° angle under the bird's chest feathers and into the muscle beneath.

To prevent overinjecting one spot on your bird's chest, think of the chest muscle as the face of a clock and rotate injections around the clock. Start at twelve o'clock, then give the next injection at one o'clock and so on. While you're giving the injections to your pet, remain calm and talk to your bird in a soothing voice.

TOPICAL MEDICATION

Topical medications are applied directly to part of a bird's body, such as his eyes, his feet or legs, or into his nares. Have your veterinarian describe the amount of medicine you should apply, how frequently, and when you should expect to see improvement in your bird's condition.

Bandage, Splint and Collar Care

Injured birds often need to have bandages, splints or collars applied to them to aid in the healing process. If they are applied properly, these devices can help support and protect injured muscles, ligaments, tendons or bones. They can also help prevent a bird from picking at a wound with his beak. However, if any of these devices is applied improperly, it can cause serious injury. For this reason, only an avian veterinarian should place a bandage, splint or collar on your bird.

If your bird has to wear a bandage, splint or collar, here are a few points to remember:

• Keep it dry! A wet splint or bandage can cause an infection and delay healing. If the bandage or splint becomes wet, contact your veterinarian's office for an appointment to have the bandage or splint replaced.

• Watch your bird for signs of picking. Light "preening" of a bandage is normal, but digging and tearing at the dressing are not.

• If part of the bandage becomes loose or slips, the entire bandage will probably need to be changed. Contact your veterinarian's office for further instructions.

• If toes or wing tips are exposed below the bandage, check them daily for swelling. If you see swelling, the bandage could be applied too tightly and will need to be changed. Alert your veterinarian to any signs of swelling immediately.

Monitor Your Sick Bird

Although you need to observe your pet bird daily, you will need to be even more vigilant when your bird is sick. Pay attention to the number, size, color and consistency of your bird's droppings. Listen to his breathing and report any abnormalities (forced breathing, tail bobbing, gasping) to your veterinarian promptly. Watch how much food and water your bird consumes while he is sick, and weigh him daily. Check your bird's body temperature by watching to see if he huddles on the cage floor with his feathers fluffed (which means it's too cold) or sits up tall with his wings away from his body and breathes heavily (which means it's too warm). Finally, keep an eye on your bird's appearance. Is he grooming himself and sitting fairly upright, or is he hunched over and listless in a corner of his cage? If you suspect that your bird's condition has deteriorated or you do not see adequate improvement, contact your veterinarian immediately.

At-Home Care Tips

When your pet bird is recuperating from a serious illness or injury, the following tips can help you better cope with the recovery period.

First, be patient with your pet. He may be clumsy because of bandages or splints, or he may need more attention from you because he doesn't feel well. He may require hand-feeding or some other type of special diet during his recovery, or he may need to be medicated several times a day. If possible, have all members of your family get involved in caring for your recuperating pet—your family's relationship with your pet will benefit from everyone's involvement, and one person won't become worn out or overly stressed because he or she had to perform all the nursing care.

You should also expect to have a change in your routine while your bird is recovering. You may find yourself losing sleep because you're sitting up with your pet, or you may have to alter some of your social calendar to accommodate medication times. You may also want to come home for lunch to check on your pet, or you may need to arrange to work from home for a few days when your bird first comes home from your avian veterinarian's office. Discuss any potential schedule changes with your avian veterinarian before you bring your bird home from the clinic to ensure that your bird's needs will be met during his recovery.

Next, keep your avian veterinarian's number handy, and don't be afraid to use it. Your avian veterinarian and his or her support staff can answer any routine questions you may have during your bird's recovery, and you will need to alert them promptly to any sudden changes in your bird's activity level, appetite or appearance.

Check on your bird regularly during his recuperation, and give him attention immediately if he needs it. Some birds may learn to exploit their recuperation and may beg for attention long after they've recovered, but most will appreciate the attention given to them by caring owners when they aren't feeling well.

While your bird is recuperating, you may have to make some adjustments to his cage. You may have to lower or remove perches to accommodate your bird's ability to move around his cage, and you may want to lower some toys to make it easier for him to play while he's recovering.

Focus on Prevention

Taking proactive steps to safeguard your bird's health may prevent your bird from needing first aid.

The old adage, "An ounce of prevention is worth a pound of cure," certainly holds true for avian medicine. Many serious illnesses can be prevented when owners feed their pet birds balanced diets, keep their pets' cages scrupulously clean and take their birds to an avian veterinarian for regular examinations.

Your avian veterinarian can be a valuable ally when it comes to keeping your pet bird healthy. He or she can answer questions about avian nutrition and health, and he or she can also help you better understand your bird's behavior. Your avian veterinarian can help you groom your bird's wings and nails to protect him from injury or escape, and your avian veterinarian's office may even provide a home away from home for your pet bird while you are on vacation.

Select your avian veterinarian before you even bring your bird home and start forming an alliance with the doctor to ensure your bird's good health as soon as possible—ideally on your way home from the breeder or pet store with your new feathered friend.

In some cases, avian emergencies can be eliminated or seriously reduced by using some caution and common sense. For example, if you put your bird back in his cage before you start to prepare supper, your pet can't fall in the soup pot and be burned, and he can't nibble on the chocolate cake you made for dessert, which may poison him. If you don't allow your bird out of his cage when your Labrador Retriever is in the house, your dog can't step on your pet bird and injure him. If you make arrangements to board your bird while your home is being fumigated, he won't be overcome by fumes from the chemicals used to kill the termites.

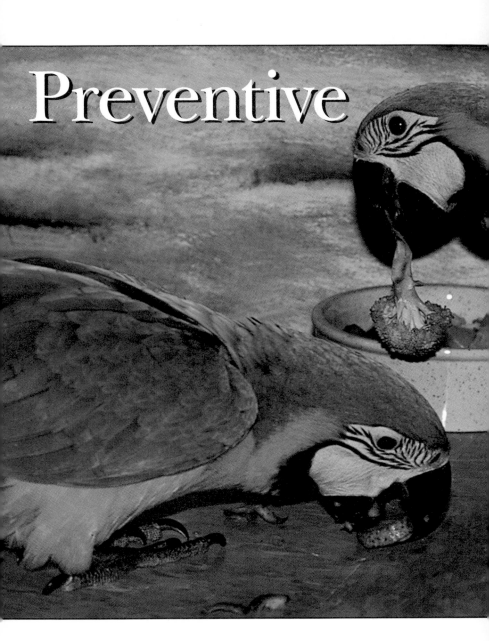

Preventive

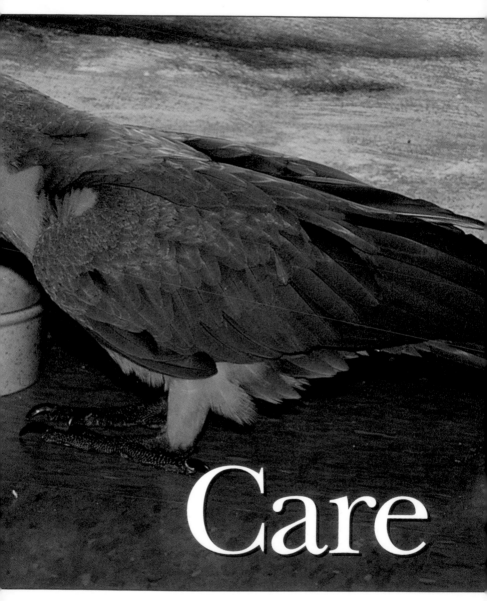

part two

Care

chapter 4

Your Bird's
Nutrition

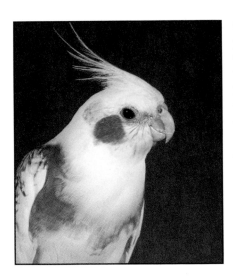

Good nutrition is the most important element in the health, vitality and longevity of pet birds. However, many birds have traditionally been fed little more than seeds and water. Think about how dull and unhealthy it would be for you to eat only one type of food—it isn't any more interesting for your pet bird. An inadequate diet causes a number of health problems, some of which require emergency care to resolve.

Vitamins and Minerals

Pet birds require about a dozen vitamins—A, D, E, K, B_1, B_2, niacin, B_6, B_{12}, pantothenic acid, biotin, folic acid and choline—to stay healthy, but they can only partially manufacture D_3 and niacin. A balanced diet can help provide the rest.

Along with the vitamins listed above, pet birds need trace amounts of some minerals to maintain good health. These minerals are calcium, phosphorus, sodium, chlorine, potassium, magnesium, iron, zinc, copper, sulphur, iodine and manganese. A well-balanced diet should provide your bird with these nutrients.

When you bring your pet bird home, be sure to bring along the same kind of food the bird was eating at the breeder's or at the pet store. This will help ease your pet's transition to her new home, and it will also help ensure her good health.

Many pet birds today eat pelleted diets, which provide balanced nutrition. If, however, your pet's diet consists of mostly fresh foods and seeds, you may want to sprinkle a good-quality vitamin-and-mineral powder onto the fresh foods, where it has the best chance of sticking to the food and being eaten. Vitamin-enriched seed diets may provide some supplementation, but some of them add the vitamins and minerals to the seed hull, which your pet will discard while she's eating. Avoid adding vitamin and mineral supplements to your bird's water dish, because they can act as a growth medium for bacteria. They may also cause the water to taste different to your bird, which may discourage her from drinking.

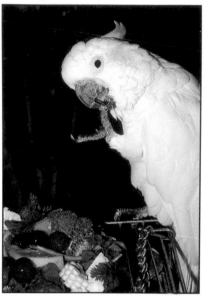

A well-balanced diet will help keep your bird free of respiratory infections, poor feather condition, flaky skin and reproductive problems.

A Balanced Diet

Ideally, your pet bird's diet should contain equal parts of pellets, grain and legumes, and dark green or dark orange vegetables and fruits. You can supplement these foods with small amounts of well-cooked meat or eggs, or dairy products,

GRAINS AND LEGUMES

The grain and legumes portion of your bird's diet can include a pelleted or formulated diet. Pelleted diets are created by mixing as many as forty different nutrients into a mash and then forcing (or extruding) the hot mixture through a machine to form various shapes. Some pelleted diets have colors and flavors added, while others are fairly plain.

These formulated diets provide balanced nutrition for your pet bird in an easy-to-serve form that reduces the amount of wasted food and eliminates the chance for a bird to pick through a smorgasbord of healthy foods to find her favorites and reject the foods she isn't particularly fond of. Some birds accept pelleted diets quickly, while others require some persuading.

To help your pet convert to a pelleted diet, offer pellets alongside of or mixed in with her current diet. Once you see that your bird is eating the pellets, begin to gradually increase the amount of pellets you offer at mealtime while decreasing the amount of other food you serve. Within a couple of weeks, your bird should be eating her pellets with gusto!

If your pet bird seems a bit finicky about trying pellets, another bird in the house may show your reluctant eater how yummy pellets can be, or you may have to act as if you are enjoying the pellets as a snack in front of your pet. Really play up your apparent enjoyment of this new food because it will pique your bird's curiosity and make the pellets exceedingly interesting to your pet.

Another conversion method you may want to try is to offer your bird a dish of pellets for her morning meal, then offer her regular diet of seeds and fresh foods for

CONVERTING BIRDS TO PELLETS

The following suggestions may be useful for owners who want to convert their pets from seed-based to pelleted diets:

1. Offer pellets in gradually increasing amounts in the current diet while decreasing the amount of seeds being fed. Offer pellets either whole or pulverized to tempt your bird into trying them.

2. Offer only pellets to your bird in the morning, while offering the old diet in the evening.

3. Flavor pellets with sauces, juices, soups or broths to make them more palatable.

her evening meal. Some hungry birds will dive right into the bowl of pellets, while others may take a few servings to learn what this new item is and that it's good to eat.

If your bird seems reluctant to try pellets, you can soak them in sauces, juices, soups or broths to make them more appealing to your pet.

Finally, owners who want to convert their pet birds to pelleted diets may have to employ a little "tough love" during the conversion process, especially if the bird seems unwilling to eat. Keep in mind that very few healthy birds will willingly starve themselves. However, many pet birds can and do manipulate their owners by refusing to eat until a favorite food is offered. Ask your avian veterinarian for more hints on how to convert your pet bird to a pelleted diet.

A varied diet is an important part of keeping your bird emotionally and physically healthy.

Although a bird can eat a pellet-only diet and maintain her health, it's wise to offer your bird some variety in her food bowl. By giving her a variety of healthful foods to choose from, you allow your pet to make some choices about her life and exercise some control over her day-to-day routine.

In the wild, birds make choices all day long about where to forage, eat, sleep and play, but in captivity, many of those choices are made for them. This leaves them with a lot of time on their hands and a lot of energy to expend—time and energy that can quickly be channeled into destructive behaviors if constructive alternatives aren't offered.

SEEDS

Seeds have a limited role in a pet bird's diet: They should be offered as an occasional treat or as a training reward. Although seeds have been traditionally offered as a large part of a pet bird's diet, they lack many important vitamins and minerals pet birds need to maintain their health.

SPROUTING SEEDS

Some birds enjoy their seed treats more if the seeds are sprouted. To sprout seeds, you will need to soak them overnight in lukewarm water. Drain the water off and let the seeds sit in a closed cupboard or other out-of-the-way place for twenty-four hours. Rinse the sprouted seeds thoroughly before offering them to your bird. If the seeds don't sprout, they aren't fresh, and you'll need to find another source for your bird's food.

FRUITS AND VEGETABLES

Dark green or dark orange vegetables and fruits contain vitamin A, which is an important part of a bird's diet that is not supplied by most grains, legumes and seeds. This vitamin helps fight off infection and keeps a bird's eyes, mouth and respiratory system healthy. Some vitamin-A-rich foods are carrots, yams, sweet potatoes, broccoli, dried red peppers, dandelion greens and spinach.

Fresh fruits and vegetables are healthy additions to your bird's diet.

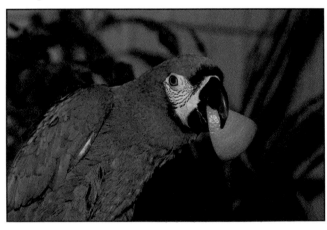

You may be wondering whether or not to offer frozen or canned vegetables and fruits to your bird. Some birds will eat frozen vegetables and fruits, while others dislike the somewhat mushy texture of these foodstuffs. The high sodium content in some canned foods may make them unhealthy for your pet. Frozen and canned foods will serve your bird's needs in an emergency, but offer only fresh foods on a regular basis.

PROTEIN

Along with small portions of well-cooked meat, you can also offer your bird bits of tofu, water-packed tuna, fully scrambled eggs, cottage cheese, unsweetened yogurt or low-fat cheese. However, use discretion with dairy products, because a bird's digestive system lacks sufficient quantities of the enzyme lactase to fully process dairy foods.

FOOD FOR HUMANS

Introduce young birds to healthy food early so that they learn to appreciate a varied diet. Some adult birds cling tenaciously to seed-only diets, which aren't as nutritious as a varied diet. Offer adult birds fresh foods, too, in the hope that they may try something new.

Regardless of the healthy fresh foods you offer your pet, be sure to remove food from the cage promptly to prevent spoilage and to help keep your bird healthy. Ideally, you should change the food in your bird's cage every two to four hours (about every thirty minutes in warm weather), so a pet bird should be all right with a tray of food to pick through in the morning, another to select from during the afternoon and a third fresh salad to nibble on for dinner.

WATER

Provide your bird with fresh, clean water once a day to maintain her good health. Change the water more frequently if you notice that your bird eliminates in her water dish or tries to make "soup" in her dish by dropping in bits of uneaten food. If your bird seems to enjoy making a mess of her water bowl, you may want to consider providing a water bottle (such as those used by rabbits or hamsters) as an additional water source.

When offering a water bottle to your pet bird, be sure she knows it's a water source before you remove her water bowl. If your pet is particularly mischievous, a water bottle may not be the complete solution to your problems because some clever birds have been known to stuff a seed into the drinking tube, which allows all the water to drain out of the bottle. This creates a thirsty bird and a soggy cage, neither of which is an ideal situation.

If your bird makes a mess of her water bowl, add a water bottle to her cage to ensure that she is well hydrated.

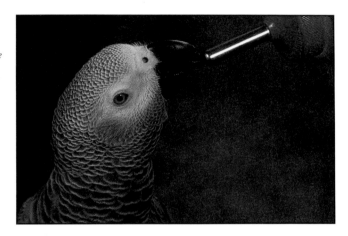

Special Diets

LORIES AND LORIKEETS

Lories and lorikeets will require a slightly different diet than other birds. These brush-tongued birds will need nectar or a special lory diet to maintain their good health, rather than seeds.

SOFTBILLED BIRDS

Diets for softbills, such as toucans, mynahs and starlings, should include a variety of fruits, some vegetables, a good source of protein and plenty of fresh water. Suitable fruit choices include apples, pears, papaya and grapes. Cut up any fruit before serving because your bird will likely swallow the food whole. Chunks of raw dark orange and green vegetables can be added to the fruit mixture to provide

---

INGREDIENTS FOR A HEALTHFUL BIRD DIET

Pellets

Cooked whole grains and legumes, such as rice, beans or pasta

Fresh vegetables

Fresh fruits in smaller amounts

Occasional treats, such as fresh seeds

---

some variety in your softbill's diet. Protein sources include commercial mynah bird pellets or insects, such as mealworms or crickets.

Pay attention to the iron content of foods you offer your softbills because some birds can develop iron storage disease, in which high levels of iron accumulate in the bird's liver. Limit the iron content in your softbill's diet to less than 150 parts per million. Foods with high iron contents to avoid include commercial dog and cat foods, monkey biscuits, raisins and other dried fruits and spinach. Some softbills require nectar as a primary part of their diet, while others enjoy it as an occasional treat.

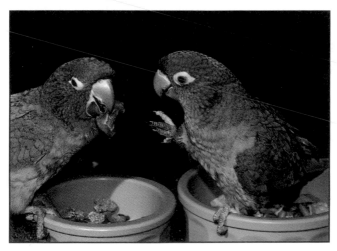

Food and water cups should be washed frequently, especially if your birds like to sit in them.

Foods to Avoid

Foods that are harmful to pet birds are alcohol, rhubarb, avocado (the skin and the area around the pit can be toxic), as well as highly salted, sweetened or fatty foods. You should avoid giving your pet chocolate, because it contains a chemical, theobromine, that birds cannot digest as completely as people can. Chocolate can kill your bird, so resist the temptation to share this treat with your pet. You will also want to avoid giving her seeds or pits from apples, apricots, cherries, peaches, pears and plums, because they can be harmful to your pet's health.

Let common sense be your guide in choosing which foods can be offered to your bird: If it's healthy for you, it's probably okay to share. However, remember to reduce the size of the portion you offer to your bird—a smaller bird-sized portion will be more appealing to your pet than a larger, human-sized portion.

Show your affection by stroking your bird—kissing is hazardous for her health.

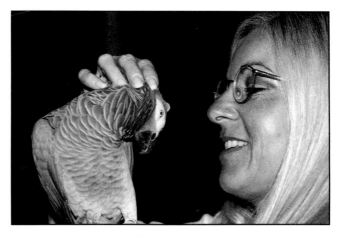

TAKE CARE WITH KISSES

Don't kiss your pet bird on the beak (kiss her on top of her head instead) or allow your bird to put her head into your mouth, nibble on your lips or preen your teeth. Although you may see birds doing this on television or in pictures in a magazine and think that it's a cute trick, it's really unsafe for your bird's health and well-being. Also, the friendliest of birds have been known to bite their owners on the lips without any provocation whatsoever from the owner. These bites hurt and can require stitches or plastic surgery to repair.

While sharing healthy food with your bird is completely acceptable, sharing something that you've already taken a bite of is not. The bacteria in human saliva are perfectly normal for people but are potentially toxic to birds, so please don't share partially eaten food with your pet. Make certain that guests and other family members know not to share their food with your bird. Because feeding a bird is so much fun for children, monitor them closely so that they don't break this rule. For your bird's health and your peace of mind, give a separate portion or plate.

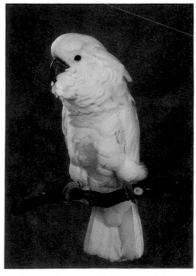

Household Hazards

The phrase "curiosity killed the cat" could easily be rewritten to reflect a pet bird's curious nature. Birds seem to be able to get into just about anything, which means they can get themselves into potentially dangerous situations rather quickly. Because of this natural curiosity, pet bird owners must be extremely vigilant when their birds are out of their cages.

Part of this vigilance should include bird-proofing your home. Remember that some of the larger parrots are intellectually on a similar level as a toddler. You wouldn't let a toddler have free run of your house without taking a few precautions to safeguard the child from harm, and you should extend the same concern to your pet birds.

Safe Cage Concerns

Your bird's cage must be large enough to house your bird as well as his food and water bowls, perches and toys. Select the largest cage that you can provide, because your bird needs space to feel comfortable. Remember, too, that parrots and softbills like flying across an area, rather than hovering up and down. For this reason, long rectangular cages that offer horizontal space for short flights are preferred to tall cages that don't provide much flying room.

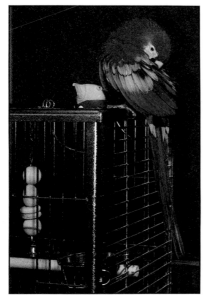

Choose a cage that has plenty of room for your bird to move about, as well as adequate space for food and water bowls, perches and toys.

Don't try to recycle cages that have been used for rabbits or other small animals when housing your bird. In many cases, these cages are made from galvanized wire. If the bird gets bored and chews on the cage wire, he may consume enough of the galvanized finish to get zinc poisoning.

Parrots should not be housed in wooden or bamboo cages unless the wood or bamboo is lined with wire or wire mesh. A busy parrot beak will destroy a wooden or bamboo cage, and you'll be left with the problem of finding a new cage for your pet. These cages are designed for finches and other songbirds that are less likely than a parrot to chew on their homes.

CAGE FINISH

Examine the cage finish carefully before making your final selection. Make sure that it is not chipped, bubbled or peeling, because a curious bird may find the spot and continue removing the finish. This can cause a cage to look old and worn before its time, and some cages may start to rust without their protective finishes, which can mean that a cage needs repainting or replacement before its time. Finally, if your pet ingests any of the finish, he could become ill.

BAR SPACING

Reject any cage that has bar spacing that is too wide for your pet bird; he may escape through the wider bars or he may get stuck between the bars and injure himself. The recommended sizes of the bar spacing for commonly kept pet birds follow: canaries, finches, budgies and lovebirds, ³/₈ inch; cockatiels and small conures, ½ to ³/₄ inch; Amazons, African greys and other medium-sized parrots, ³/₄ to 1 inch; macaws and cockatoos, ³/₄ to 1½ inches.

Do not choose a cage that has sharp interior wires because they could poke your bird. Birds may injure themselves on ornate decorative scrollwork on the cage. Additionally, make sure the cage you choose has some horizontal bars in it for your bird to climb and exercise on.

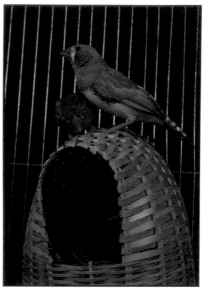

CAGE DOOR

Investigate the different types of doors on the cages you are considering for your bird. Does the door open easily for you, yet remain secure enough to keep your bird in his cage when you close the door? Is it wide enough for you to get your hand in and out of the cage comfortably? Will your bird's food bowl or a bowl of bath water fit through it easily? Does the door open up, down or to the side? Some bird owners prefer that their pets have a play porch on a door that opens drawbridge style, while others are happy with doors that open to the side.

Prevent escape and injury by choosing a cage with bars that are spaced apart appropriately for your bird's size.

PERCHES

Another important factor to consider when selecting a cage is the type of perches that come with the cage. Keep in mind that your bird spends most of his time on his feet. You can help prevent foot problems by purchasing appropriate-sized perches for your bird when you choose the cage.

Try to buy two different diameters or materials so your bird's feet won't get tired of standing on the same-sized perch of the same material day after day. Think of how tired your feet would feel if you stood barefoot on a piece of wood all day, then imagine how it would feel to stand barefoot on that piece of wood every day for ten or fifteen years. Sounds pretty uncomfortable, doesn't it? That's basically what your bird has to look forward to if you don't vary his perching choices.

Recommended perch diameters are as follows: $\frac{3}{8}$ inch for finches and canaries, $\frac{1}{2}$ inch for budgies, $\frac{5}{8}$ inch for cockatiels, $\frac{3}{4}$ inch for conures, 1 inch for Amazons and other medium-sized parrots and 2 inches for cockatoos and macaws.

Try to buy one perch at the recommended size for your bird, and a slightly larger perch to give your pet a chance to stretch his foot muscles. Birds spend almost all of their lives standing, so keeping their feet healthy is important. Also, avian foot problems are much easier to prevent than they are to treat.

Types of Perches

You'll probably notice a lot of different kinds of perches when you visit your pet store. Along with the traditional wooden dowels, bird owners can now purchase perches made from manzanita branches, PVC tubes and rope to terra-cotta or concrete grooming perches.

Manzanita offers birds varied diameters on the same perch, along with chewing possibilities, while a PVC perch is almost indestructible. (Make sure any PVC perches you offer your bird have been scuffed slightly with sandpaper to improve traction on the perch.) Rope perches also offer varied diameters and a softer perching surface than wood or plastic perches. Terra-cotta and concrete perches provide slightly abrasive surfaces that birds can use to groom their beaks without severely damaging the skin on their feet in the process. Some birds suffer foot abrasions by standing on these perches; watch your pet carefully for signs of sore feet (an inability to perch or climb, favoring a foot or raw, sore skin on the feet) if you choose to use these perches in your pet's cage. If your bird shows signs of lameness, remove the abrasive perches immediately and arrange for your avian veterinarian to examine your bird.

Do not use sandpaper covers on perches. These sleeves, touted as nail-trimming devices, really do little to trim a bird's nails. Sandpaper perch covers abrade the surface of your bird's feet, which can leave them vulnerable to infections and can make moving about the cage painful for your pet.

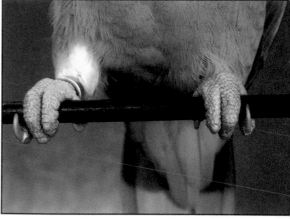

When placing perches in your bird's cage, try to vary the heights slightly so your bird has different "levels" in his cage. Don't place any perches over food or water dishes, because birds can and will contaminate food or water by eliminating in it. Finally, place one perch higher than the rest for a nighttime sleeping roost. Pet birds like to sleep on the highest point they can find to perch, so don't forget to provide this security for your pet.

This parrot's perch is too small. Choose perches that are the appropriate size or larger for your bird so that your pet can exercise his foot muscles.

CAGE TRAY

When you are looking at a cage, don't forget to examine the cage tray. Remember that you will be changing the paper in this tray at least once a day for the rest of your bird's life. Does the tray slide in and out of the cage easily? Is the tray an odd shape or size? Will you need to cut paper into unusual shapes to fit in the tray, or will paper towels, newspapers or clean sheets of used computer paper fit easily? The easier it is to remove and reline, the more likely you will be to change the lining of the tray daily. Can the cage tray be replaced if it becomes damaged and unusable? Ask your pet store staff or the cage manufacturer's customer service department before making your purchase.

HOUSEHOLD HAZARDS

Some household hazards outside your bird's cage to be aware of include:

- unscreened windows and doors

- mirrors

- exposed electrical cords

- toxic houseplants

- unattended ashtrays

- venetian blind cords

- sliding glass doors

- ceiling fans

- open washing machines, dryers, refrigerators, freezers, ovens or dishwashers

- open toilet bowls

- uncovered fish tanks

- leaded stained glass items or inlaid jewelry

- uncovered cooking pots on the stove

- crayons and permanent markers

- pesticides, rodent killers and snail bait

- untended stove burners

- candles

- open trash cans

Clean black-and-white newsprint, paper towels or sheets of printing paper are the best choices of cage substrate. Sand, ground corncobs or walnut shells may be sold by your pet supply store, but they make poor choices for cage flooring material because they tend to hide droppings and discarded food quite well. This can cause a bird owner to forget to change the cage tray on the principle that if it doesn't look dirty, it must not be dirty. This can result in a thriving, robust colony of bacteria in the bottom of the bird's cage, which can quickly lead to a sick bird. Newsprint and other paper products don't hide the dirt; in fact, they seem to draw attention to it, which leads conscientious bird owners to keep their pets' homes scrupulously clean.

CAGE FLOOR

The floor of the cage you've chosen should have a grille that will keep your bird out of the debris that falls to the bottom of the cage, such as droppings, seed hulls, molted feathers and discarded food. The grille will help to ensure your pet's long-term good health. Having something between the cage and the tray also makes it easier to keep your pet bird in his cage while you're cleaning the cage tray.

Bird-Proofing

Eliminating potential problems and maintaining healthful conditions in your home and your bird's cage will prevent most health problems. Before you buy your bird, go through each room in your house and take care of as many foreseeable problems as possible.

INSPECT EACH ROOM

A pet bird should be taken out of his cage to interact with the family and to explore his surroundings under close supervision every day. As a conscientious owner, you need to realize that potential hazards to your pet's health exist in almost every room of your home and take steps to protect your pet from harm. The following list will inform you of the potentially dangerous situations that can happen in each room, so you can take action to prevent accidents.

Kitchen

The kitchen is a popular spot for birds and their owners to hang out, especially around mealtime. It is also the most dangerous room in the house for a pet bird. Put your bird back in his cage during meal preparation to protect him from flying or falling into the trash can or from climbing into an appliance and getting trapped.

If you're going to let your pet out of his cage when you're in the kitchen, keep him away from the stove because he could be seriously injured by a hot stove element, an

---

SAFE PLANTS

Some safe plants include:

Acacia
African violet
Bamboo
Begonia
Blueberry
Bougainvillea
Bromeliads
Citrus (any)
Creeping charlie
Creeping jenny
Dandelion
Eucalyptus
Ferns
Figs
Herbs (oregano, rosemary, thyme)
Hibiscus
Magnolia
Mango
Manzanita
Marigold
Nasturtium
Nectarine
Papaya
Pear
Plum
Prune
Raspberry
Rose
Rosemary
Thyme

uncovered pot of boiling water or a sizzling frying pan on the stove. As you prepare the meal, share only healthy foods with your bird—no chocolate, avocado or rhubarb.

One of the biggest hazards faced by pet birds is the fumes emitted by overheated nonstick cookware or other items treated with nonstick coating, including bakeware, drip pans, cookie sheets, waffle irons, irons and ironing board covers. Polytetrafluoroethylene or PTFE, the polymer that covers nonstick cookware, produces fumes that are extremely toxic to birds when it is heated above 530° F. Nonstick cookware is not recommended for bird-owning households because of the health risk it poses to pet birds.

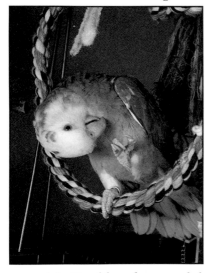

Your bird should spend some time out of his cage, under your close supervision, every day.

Bathroom

The bathroom can be a fun place to spend time with your bird as you prepare for work or for an evening out, but you have to supervise him at all times. Don't let him chew on the cord of your blow dryer, and don't use products with strong fumes, such as perfume, hairspray or cleaning products, if your pet is in the room. Protect your bird from illness by storing jewelry and prescription or over-the-counter medication out of your bird's reach.

Living Room

For your bird's safety and the well-being of your valuables, supervise your bird at all times when he is out of his cage. Don't let him play in the sofa cushions—he could become trapped between them. Also, don't let family members leave the screen door open because your pet could escape through the open door.

Keep television remote controls and other interesting chewable items out of your pet's reach, too, or you may find yourself without all of the buttons on your remote control! Offer your bird safe chew toys to play with as you watch TV together in the evenings.

Home Office

Your home office can be like a playground for birds, but you'll have to be on your toes to keep your pet from harming himself. Don't let him chew or get tangled in computer cords; nibble on potentially poisonous markers, glue sticks or crayons; or impale himself on push pins. You may find that it is best to have your pet sit on a portable perch complete with food cup and safe bird toys when he visits you in your home office.

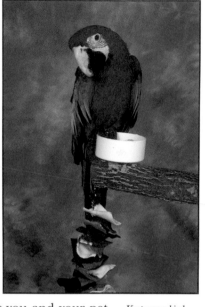

Home Workshop

Birds like to be where their owners are, so if you're a handy person, you and your bird may spend a lot of time in the home workshop. If you do, make sure that a securely screened window is open to provide adequate ventilation for you and your pet, and to keep your bird away from paints, thinners, glues or other chemicals stored in the workshop. Also watch him to make sure that he does not injure himself on tools found there.

Keep your bird safe when he's out of his cage by providing him with a portable perch to play on.

You can put your bird's travel cage or carrier to good use when you're in the home workshop. Your bird can still see you and be close to you, but he'll be protected from harm.

Garage

Be careful when taking your bird into the garage because he could be overcome by carbon monoxide fumes from your car, especially if the garage door is closed. Also be aware that some birds are afraid of the dark and may act up if you take them into the garage without turning the lights on right away.

Although there are many household hazards that you need to be aware of, you should not keep your bird locked up in his cage all the time. All birds, especially parrots, need time out of their cages to maintain physical and mental health. Simply be aware of some of the dangers that may exist in your home and pay attention to your bird's behavior so you can intervene before he becomes ill or injured.

TOXIC HOUSEHOLD PRODUCTS

Did you know that among other toxic items, the following household products are poisonous to your bird? Read the labels of what you buy, and keep this list in mind when bird-proofing your home.

aspirin

corn and wart removers

crayons

deodorants

detergents

disinfectants

fabric softeners

hair dyes

indelible markers

insecticides

kerosene

matches

model glue

mothballs

nail polish/remover

perfume

shaving lotion

shoe polish

super glue

Protect Your Pet from Toxic Fumes

To help protect your pet from harmful chemical fumes, consider using some "green" cleaning alternatives, such as baking soda and vinegar to clear clogged drains, baking soda instead of scouring powder to clean tubs and sinks, lemon juice and mineral oil to polish furniture and white vinegar and water as a window cleaner. These simple solutions to cleaning problems often work better than higher-priced, brand-name products.

If you're considering a home improvement project, think about your bird first. Fumes from paint or formaldehyde, which can be found in carpet backing, paneling and particle board, can cause pets to become ill. Consider boarding your pet until the project is complete and the house is aired out fully. You can consider the house safe for your pet when you cannot smell any trace of any of the products used in the remodeling.

Having your home fumigated for termites or other pests poses a potentially hazardous situation to your pet. Ask your exterminator for information about the types of chemicals that will be used in your home, and inquire if pet-safe formulas, such as electrical currents or liquid nitrogen, are available. If your house must be treated chemically, arrange to board your bird at your avian veterinarian's office or with a friend before, during and after the fumigation to ensure that no harm comes to your pet. Make sure your house is aired out completely before bringing your bird home, too.

Your Bird and Other Pets

Other pets can harm your bird's health. If you have a dog, cat or more than one bird, you must supervise the time they spend interacting. Keep your bird separate from other household pets if they become aggressive. If your bird tangles with another pet in your home, contact your avian veterinarian immediately because emergency treatment (for bacterial infection from a puncture wound or shock from being stepped on or suffering a broken bone) may be required to save your bird's life.

HARMFUL PLANTS

Amaryllis

Apple (seeds)

Apricot (pits)

Avocado

Azalea

Beans (all types if uncooked)

Bulb flowers

Chrysanthemum

Daffodil

Dieffenbachia

Holly

Hydrangea

Iris (blue flag)

Ivy

Lily of the valley

Oleander

Peach (pits)

Philodendron

Poinsettia

Potato

Rhododendron

Rhubarb

Wisteria

chapter 6

Reducing
Your Pet's
Stress

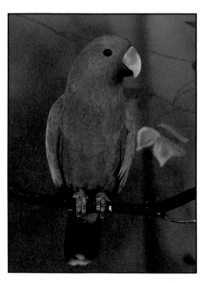

Although it's not a disease per se, stress can contribute to illness in our pet birds, just as it can cause illness in people. Stress in a bird's life can function in both good and bad ways. Positive stress produces excitement and enjoyment, such as a play session with a favored person or a ride in the car. Negative stress causes illness and behavioral problems. Negative stress can be caused by underlying tension in the home between partners or the bird feeling insecure because her cage is in the center of the room.

Ideally, your bird's life will have some combination of good stress and bad stress in it. One of your jobs as a bird owner is to try to minimize the bad stress and provide some good stress. It's impossible to remove all stresses from your bird's life, just as it's impossible to remove them from your own. However, by striking a balance, you can help your bird live a more comfortable, less stressed life.

Decreasing "Bad" Stress

To help your bird feel less stressed, provide her with a safe, secure cage in a safe, secure location in your home. This cage should have appropriate-sized bar spacing and accessories that are designed for your species of bird. It also should be located in a part of your home in which you and your family spend time regularly so your bird will feel as if she's part your daily routine. Remember that birds need to feel secure in their cages, so make sure that your bird's home has at least one solid wall behind it. This will let her relax a bit because she'll feel as though predators and other scary things won't be able to sneak up on her.

CLEAN ENVIRONMENT, HEALTHY BIRD

To keep your pet healthy, change the cage paper and food and water bowls daily (be sure to wash the bowls thoroughly with soap and water and rinse them completely), and scrub the cage every week to protect her from illness and to make her surroundings more enjoyable.

STRESSORS
Almost anything in the environment can cause your bird to become stressed. Among the common stressors for birds are:
• new people in the home
• new pets in the home
• loud noises
• sudden movements
• earthquakes
• rearrangement of furniture in the bird's room
• a stressed owner
• unclean feathers
• sexual maturity/urge to breed
• boredom (not enough toys or attention from her owner)
• feelings of insecurity
• an unbalanced diet
• lack of sleep
• loneliness

PROVIDE STIMULATION

An interesting environment will increase the good stress and decrease the bad stress for your bird. Make

93

your pet feel that she's part of your family. Entertain and challenge your bird's curiosity with a variety of safe toys. Rotate these toys in and out of your bird's cage regularly, and discard any that become soiled, broken, frayed, worn or otherwise unsafe. When you are away from home, leave a radio or television on for your bird because a too-quiet environment can be stressful for many birds.

DEVOTE TIME TO YOUR BIRD

Take your bird out of her cage for playtime on a regular basis. Let her sit on a portable perch near your family at the dinner table or perch on the arm of your recliner as you watch television in the evenings. Set up a play gym for your pet in the family room so she can spend time out of her cage playing and interacting with family members.

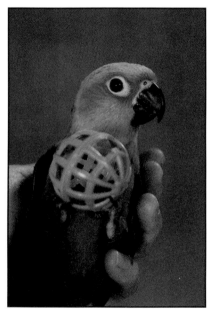

Decrease your bird's stress level by providing her with stimulating toys and one-on-one attention.

Pay attention to your pet on a consistent basis. Don't lavish abundant attention on the bird when you first bring her home and then gradually lose interest in her. Birds are sensitive, intelligent creatures that will not understand such a mixed message. Set aside a portion of each day to spend with your bird—you'll both enjoy it and your relationship will benefit from it. Besides, wasn't companionship one of the things you were looking for when you picked your bird as a pet? Just devote a little time each day to your pet bird, and soon the two of you will have formed a lifelong bond of trust and mutual enjoyment.

OFFER NUTRITIOUS FOOD

Part of providing an interesting environment is offering a healthful and interesting diet because many birds play with their food in addition to eating it. Your bird's diet should include seeds or pellets, small portions of fresh vegetables and fruits and healthy food that you eat. Provide the freshest food possible, and remove partially eaten or discarded food from the cage before it has a chance to spoil and make your pet sick. Your bird should also have access to clean, fresh drinking water at all times.

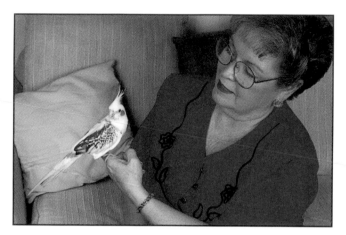

Birds like routine—try to feed, play with and put your bird to sleep close to the same time every day.

FIND AN AVIAN VETERINARIAN

Next, establish a good working relationship with a qualified avian veterinarian before you bring your bird home (preferably on your way home from the pet store or breeder). Don't wait for an emergency to locate a veterinarian.

Once you've found an excellent avian veterinarian, take your pet to the office for regular checkups, as well as when you notice a change in her routine. Illnesses in birds are sometimes difficult to detect before it's too late to save the bird, so preventive care helps head off serious problems before they develop.

KEEP A ROUTINE

Your bird will be less stressed if she can follow a routine. Make sure that she's fed at about the same time each day, her playtime out of her cage occurs regularly and that her bedtime is well established.

DON'T FORGET ABOUT BIRD-PROOFING

To ensure your bird's safety, clip her wings regularly. Bird-proof your home and practice bird safety by closing windows and doors securely before you let your bird out of her cage, keeping your bird indoors when she isn't caged and ensuring that your pet doesn't chew on anything harmful (from houseplants to leaded glass windows or lampshades to power cords) or become poisoned by toxic fumes from overheated nonstick cookware, cleaning products and other household products.

Stressful Situations

Certain situations bring their own particular types of stress to your pet bird's life.

MOLTING

Your bird may seek out your head-scratching skills when she is molting.

Molting can be a stressful event for your bird. At least once a year, your pet bird will molt, or lose her feathers. Many pet birds seem to be in a perpetual molt, with feathers falling out and coming in throughout the summer.

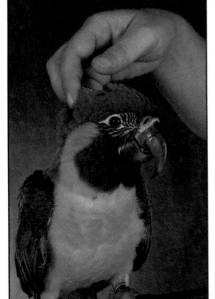

You can consider your bird in molting season when you see a lot of whole feathers in the bottom of the cage and you notice that your bird seems to have broken out in a rash of stubby little aglets (those plastic tips on the ends of your shoelaces). These are the feather sheaths, made of keratin, that help new pinfeathers break through the skin. The sheaths also help protect growing feathers from damage until the feather completes their growth cycle.

You may notice that your pet is a little more irritable during the molt; this is to be expected. Think about how you would feel if you had all these itchy new feathers coming in all of a sudden. However, your bird may actively seek out more time with you during the molt because owners are handy to have around when a bird has an itch on the top of her head that she can't quite scratch! (Scratch these new feathers gently because some of them may still be growing in and may be sensitive to the touch.) Some birds may benefit from special conditioning foods during the molt; discuss this option with your avian veterinarian.

WEATHER CHANGES

Warm weather requires a little extra vigilance on the part of a pet bird owner to ensure that your pet remains comfortable. You must also protect your pet from sunstroke or overheating. To help keep your pet cool, keep her out of the direct sun, offer her lots of fresh, juicy vegetables and fruits (be sure to remove these fresh foods from the cage promptly to prevent your bird from eating spoiled food) and mist her lightly with a clean spray bottle (filled with water only) that is used solely for birdie showers.

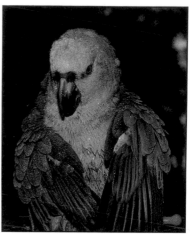

Keep your bird out of the direct sun and mist her with water to help her stay cool in warm weather.

By the same token, pay attention to your pet's needs when the weather turns cooler. You may want to use a heavier cage cover, especially if you lower the heat in your home at bedtime, or you may want to move the bird's cage to another location in your home that is warmer and less drafty.

HOLIDAYS

The holidays bring their own special set of stresses, and they can also be hazardous to your pet bird's health. Drafts from frequently opening and closing doors can have an impact on your bird's health, and the bustle of a steady stream of visitors can add to your pet's stress level (as well as your own).

Keep holiday plants, such as poinsettia, holly and mistletoe, as well as tinsel and ornaments, out of your bird's reach. Round jingle-type bells can sometimes trap a curious bird's toe, beak or tongue, so keep your bird away from these holiday decorations. Watch your pet around strings of lights, too, as both the bulbs and the cords can prove to be great temptations to curious beaks.

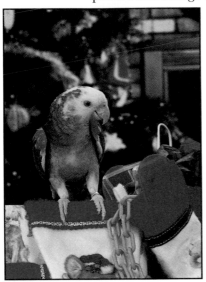

Marathon cooking sessions may result in harmful fumes for pet birds. Open the windows around your bird's cage to let in fresh air when you are cooking at high temperatures for extended periods of time. (Make sure your bird's cage is closed securely before opening a window.)

Visitors may upset your pet's routine by offering her eggnog or other rich, unhealthy treats, or by leaving a window open near your bird's cage, which could prove an

The holidays are a time when you must be extra diligent in keeping a watchful eye on your curious bird.

inviting escape route. Fumes from fireplaces or simmering pots of holiday potpourri may overcome your pet, and flickering candles or glowing embers from the hearth can tempt a pet bird right into an open flame or a serious burn.

TRAVEL

Another situation that has the potential to add bad stress to your bird's life is the stress of travel or moving. Answer the following questions before taking your bird on a trip:

- Does your bird like new adventures?
- Is there a trusted relative or friend that you can leave the bird with while you are away?
- Does your avian veterinarian's office offer boarding?
- How long will you be gone?
- Will you be visiting a foreign country?

If you are going on a family vacation, leave your bird at home in the care of a trusted friend, relative, pet sitter or avian veterinarian for two reasons. First, birds are creatures of habit that like routine, and next, taking birds across state lines or international boundaries is not without risk. It is illegal to bring some species into certain states (Quaker, or monk, parrots, for example, are believed to pose an agricultural threat in some states because of their hearty appetites), and some foreign countries have lengthy quarantine stays for pet birds.

Airline Travel

If you believe your bird would enjoy traveling and you want to take her along on a trip with you, you'll need to make some preparations before you start your trip. First, you'll need to decide how you're traveling. If you'll be flying to your destination, you'll need to make reservations for yourself and

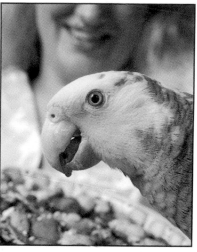

your bird. In some cases, the bird can fly with you in the passenger cabin, while in others, she will have to fly as cargo. If your bird must travel as cargo, make arrangements for direct flights and fly on the same plane as your pet. Pick up your pet promptly at the end of your journey.

You bird will probably be more comfortable and less stressed if you leave her at home with a trusted pet sitter when you travel.

Car Travel

If you'll be traveling by car, you'll need to pack some items for your pet, including a first aid kit for any accidents or emergencies along the way. In addition to the first aid kit, take along an adequate supply of your bird's food, as well as a jug or two of the water your bird is used to drinking. Your bird will be able to handle the stress of moving better if she has familiar food and water to eat and drink along the way.

You may also need to acclimate your bird to traveling in the car. Some pet birds take to this new adventure immediately, while others become so stressed out by the trip that they become carsick. Patience and persistence are usually the keys to success if your pet falls into the latter category.

To get your bird used to riding in the car, start by taking her cage (with door and cage tray well secured) out to your car and placing it inside. Make sure that your car is cool before you do this, because your pet can suffer heatstroke if you place her in a hot car and leave her there.

When your bird seems comfortable sitting in her cage in your car, take her for a short drive, such as around the block. If your bird seems to enjoy the ride (she eats, sings, whistles, talks and generally acts like nothing is wrong), then you have a willing traveler on your hands. If she seems distressed by the ride (she sits on the floor of her cage shaking, screams or vomits), then you have a bit of work ahead. Distressed birds often only need to be "taught" that car travel can be fun. You can do this by talking to your bird throughout the trip. Praise her for good behavior and reassure her that everything will be fine. Offer special treats and juicy fruits (grapes, apples or citrus fruit) so that your pet will eat and will also take in water. (On long trips, you may want to remove your pet's water dish during travel to avoid spillage. If you do take out the dish, make sure to stop frequently and give your bird water so she doesn't dehydrate.)

As your bird becomes accustomed to car travel, gradually increase the length of the trips. When your bird is comfortable with car rides, begin to condition her for the trip by packing your car as you would on departure day. If, for example, you plan to place duffel bags near your bird's cage, put the bags and the cage in the back of the car for a "practice run" before you actually begin the move so your bird can adjust to the size, shape and color of the bags. A little planning on your part will result in a well-adjusted avian traveler and a reduced stress level for you both.

If you will be traveling to another state, you will probably need to make hotel or motel reservations along the way. As you do, ask if the hotel or motel allows pets.

(The Auto Club guidebooks and other guides often provide this information, but it doesn't hurt to check the policy as you're making reservations.) Ask for non-smoking rooms to keep you and your bird healthy, and be prepared to clean up after your pet at the hotel or motel, because this will make it easier for bird owners who come after you to keep their pets in their rooms.

While you're on the road, do not leave your pet bird alone in the car because she can become overheated quickly. She can also be stolen by a passerby. Be sure not to advertise the fact that you own a pet bird to strangers you meet along the way because they might want to steal your pet, too.

Before you leave on your trip, make a final appointment with your bird's veterinarian. Have the bird evaluated, and ask for a health certificate (this may come in handy when crossing state lines).

Planning for Disaster

Disasters can be the ultimate stress-producing event for both pets and people. They can strike at any time and in any place, from earthquakes in California to ice storms in the Northeast. To ensure that you and your bird can ride out the storm, make sure that you have the following items on hand:

- three to five days' worth of canned food per person and per pet
- manual can opener
- paper plates and plastic utensils
- two gallons of water per person per day (at least three days' worth)
- portable radio and extra batteries
- flashlights and extra batteries in each room of your house
- tarps and blankets
- warm clothing and comfortable shoes
- work gloves

- first aid kits for people and for pets
- cash and coins to purchase supplies and make phone calls

Other items to consider in your disaster preparedness kit include a portable generator, a cellular phone and an ample number of carriers in which to transport your pets.

Be aware that Red Cross shelters do not accept pets under normal conditions (assistance animals are the exception), so you may have to make arrangements for you and your pet to stay elsewhere if a disaster leaves you homeless.

The Humane Society of the United States and the American Red Cross have prepared a brochure titled "Pets and Disaster: Get Prepared." To order a copy, send a self-addressed, stamped business-size envelope to The Humane Society of the United States, 2100 L St. NW, Washington, DC 20037.

chapter 7

Observing
Your Pet Bird
Daily

Being an observant owner is one of
the easiest ways you can maintain
your bird's health. It is very important
to know your bird's normal routine—
how much he eats, how often he
eliminates, when he rests and when
he plays—and report any changes to
your avian veterinarian immediately.
(When you leave your bird in the care
of a pet sitter, describe your bird's
normal routine to that person so he
or she can detect any abnormalities
quickly.)

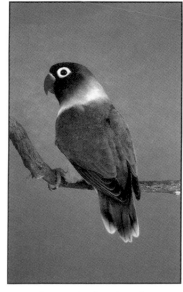

Daily Observations

Observe your pet on a daily basis
for any of the following changes in
his routine. Report any changes to your avian veterinarian immediately.

Keep track of your bird's daily routine—if there is a change in his activity level or physical appearance, contact your veterinarian immediately.

- Changes in activity that include a decrease in activity, a bird that sings or talks less, a bird that sleeps more or a bird that demonstrates decreased responsiveness to various stimuli.

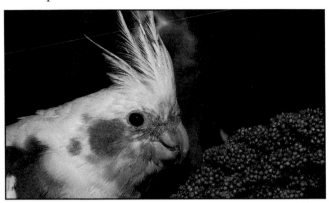

- Changes in appearance that include ruffled feathers, weakness, an inability to perch, a bird that remains on the cage floor, bleeding, injuries, convulsions or a distended abdomen.

- Breathing problems that include noisy breathing (wheezing, panting or clicking), heavy breathing (shortness of breath, open-mouthed breathing, tail bobbing), nasal discharge, a swollen area around the bird's eye or a loss of voice.

- Digestive problems including vomiting and/or regurgitation, diarrhea (it may include blood, mucus or whole seeds) or straining to eliminate.

- Musculoskeletal problems including lameness, drooping wings or a change in posture.

- Eye problems including swollen or pasted-shut eyelids, increased blinking, eye discharge, eyeball cloudiness, squinting or rubbing of the eye or the side of the face.

- Skin problems including lumps, bumps, excessive flaking of skin or beak, or overgrown beak or nails.

- Feather problems including a prolonged molt, a bird that picks at or chews his feathers or damaged (broken, crushed, twisted or deformed) feathers.

- Changes in food or water intake including a loss of appetite, a loss of weight, a decrease in food and water consumption, dehydration or an increase in food and water consumption.

- Changes in the bird's droppings in terms of amount, consistency or color.

A "HANDS-OFF" EXAMINATION

You should also perform a "hands-off" examination of your bird each day. This requires that you observe the bird, his cage and his food and water bowls daily with the following questions in mind.

Examine the Bird

- Is there anything out of the ordinary?
- Has any routine changed?
- Are the bird's eating and drinking habits normal?
- Is the bird's level of vocalizing/singing/talking about the same?

Examine the Cage

- Is the food being eaten?
- Is the water being drunk?
- Are any objects in the cage missing or chewed?
- Is there anything unusual in the cage?

Examine the Cage Floor

- Are the droppings normal?
- Are there any feathers or blood on the floor?

SIGNS OF ILLNESS

Abdominal enlargement

Bald spots in the feathers

Bleeding from the mouth

Changes in appetite or thirst

Changes in behavior, responsiveness or coordination

Discharge or swelling from the ear

Drooping wings

Labored breathing

Lameness

Lumps, bumps, bruises or cuts

Matted feathers around the vent

Noisy breathing

Overgrown nails or beaks

Plugged nares

Postural changes

Seizures

Shortness of breath

Stiffness in the joints

Swelling of or below the eyes

Unequal pupil size

Unusual eye movements

Vomiting/regurgitation

Weakness or inability to move

White deposits at the corners of the beak or on the legs

White spots in the mouth

Examine the Dishes

- Is the food bowl full of uneaten seed?

- Is the water clean?

MONITOR YOUR BIRD'S DROPPINGS

Although it may seem unpleasant to discuss, your bird's droppings require daily monitoring because they can tell you a lot about his general health. Parrot droppings are made up of fecal material, urine and urates. Fecal material is the unusable solid waste material from the bird's food. The fecal material should be tubular and form into a coil. Color can range from dark green to near black in birds that eat primarily seeds, while a brownish color is more common in birds that eat a pelleted diet. Urine is the clear liquid portion. Birds that eat a diet containing a lot of fruits and vegetables will produce more urine than birds that eat pellets or seeds. Urates, or uric acid, comprise the white or cream-colored part that often surrounds the feces.

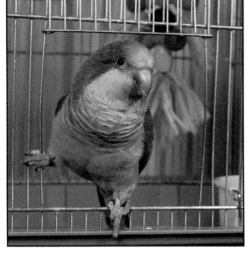

Besides monitoring your bird's general health and well-being, check his cage every day to confirm that he is eating and drinking.

Texture and consistency, along with frequency or lack of droppings, can let you know how your pet is feeling. For example, if a bird eats a lot of fruits and vegetables, his droppings are generally looser and more watery than a bird that eats primarily pellets. But watery droppings can also indicate illness, such as infection, kidney problems or occasionally diabetes, which causes a bird to drink more water than usual.

As part of your daily cage cleaning and observation of your feathered friend, look at his droppings carefully. Learn what is normal for your bird in terms of color, consistency and frequency, and report any changes to your avian veterinarian promptly.

Ten Steps to Better Bird Care

The following is a list of ten simple things that bird owners should do to help keep their pets healthy and safe.

First, **provide a safe, secure cage in a safe, secure location** in your home. This cage should have appropriate-sized bar spacing and accessories that are designed for your bird. It also should be located in a part of your home that you and your family spend time in regularly to help your bird feel part of your daily routine.

Next, **change the cage paper, food and water bowls daily** (be sure to wash the bowls thoroughly with soap and water and rinse them completely), and scrub the cage every week to protect your pet from illness and to make his surroundings more enjoyable for both of you.

Third, **clip your bird's wings regularly** to ensure his safety. Be particularly alert to new wing feathers that grow in following a molt. Close windows and doors securely before you let your bird out of his cage. You should also keep your bird indoors when he isn't caged and ensure that your pet doesn't chew on anything harmful or become poisoned by toxic fumes from overheated nonstick cookware, cleaning products and other household products.

Fourth, **offer your bird a varied diet** that includes seeds or pellets, small portions of fresh vegetables and fruits, and healthy people food. Provide the freshest food possible, and remove partially eaten or discarded food from the cage before it has a chance to spoil and make your pet sick. Your bird should also have access to clean, fresh drinking water at all times.

Next, **establish a good working relationship with a qualified avian veterinarian** early on in your bird ownership (preferably on your way home from the pet store or breeder). Don't wait for an emergency to locate a veterinarian.

Sixth, take your bird to the veterinarian for **regular checkups**, as well as when you notice a change in his routine. Illnesses in birds are sometimes difficult to detect before it's too late to save the bird, so preventive care helps head off serious problems before they develop.

Seventh, **maintain a routine for your pet**. Make sure he's fed at about the same time each day, playtime out of his cage occurs regularly and that his bedtime is well established.

Eighth, **provide an interesting environment for your bird**. Make him feel that he's part of your family. Entertain and challenge your bird's curiosity with a variety of safe toys. Rotate these toys in and out of your bird's cage regularly, and discard any that become soiled, broken, frayed, worn or otherwise unsafe.

Ninth, **leave a radio or television on for your bird when you are away from home**. An extremely quiet environment can be stressful for many birds, and stress can cause illness or other problems for your pet.

Finally, **pay attention to your bird on a consistent basis**. Don't lavish abundant attention on the bird when you first bring him home, then gradually lose interest in him. Birds are sensitive, intelligent creatures that will not understand mixed messages. Set aside a portion of each day to spend with your pet.

chapter 8

Pet Bird Grooming

Consistently grooming your bird's wings and nails will help protect her from accidents and injury. Trimming wings and nails on a regular basis will help reduce the chances of your bird catching or breaking her nail on a toy or on her cage, and you will also help protect her against accidentally flying into a window or a wall.

Although some people would say that a parrot's beak also needs trimming, most healthy birds that have enough chew toys seem to do a remarkable job of keeping their beaks

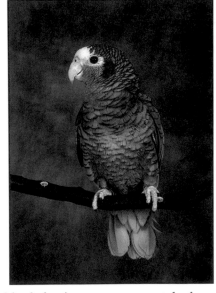

trimmed. If your bird's beak suddenly begins to overgrow, take her to your veterinarian immediately. This could be a sign of ill health.

Do not try to trim a bird's beak. A vein in the beak could easily be clipped.

Wing Trimming

The goal of a proper wing trim is to prevent your pet from flying away or flying into a window, mirror or wall while she's out of her cage. An added benefit of trimming your pet's wings is that her inability to fly well will make her more dependent on you for transportation, which should make her easier to handle. However, the bird still needs enough wing feathers so that she can glide safely to the ground if she is startled and takes flight from her cage top or play gym.

Your bird should be "toweled" and held securely to allow for safe grooming.

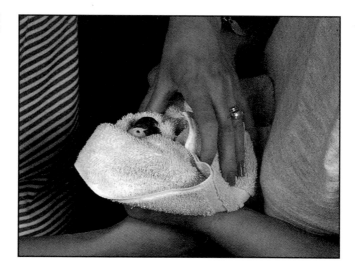

Because achieving a proper wing trim is a delicate balance, you may want to enlist the help of your avian veterinarian, at least the first time you do so. Wing trimming is a task that must be performed carefully to avoid injuring your pet, so take your time. Please ***do not*** just take up the largest pair of kitchen shears you own and start snipping away, because you could cut your bird's wing tips down to the bone in this manner.

The first step in wing feather trimming is to assemble all the things you will need and find a quiet, well-lit place to groom your pet before you catch and trim her. Your grooming tools will include:

- a well-worn washcloth or small towel to wrap your bird in

- small, sharp scissors to do the actual trimming

- needle-nosed pliers (to pull any blood feathers you may cut accidentally)

- styptic powder in case a blood feather is cut

Larger parrots require an assistant trimmer to hold the bird while the trimmer clips the wing feathers, but some birds (such as parakeets or finches) are small enough for one experienced person to handle.

Groom your pet in a quiet, well-lit place because grooming excites some birds and causes them to become wiggly. Having good light to work under will make your job easier, and having a quiet work area may just calm down your pet and make her a bit easier to handle.

> ### ABOUT COCKATIELS
>
> Cockatiels are among the fastest-flying pet birds. Their sleek, slender bodies give them an advantage over chunkier-bodied birds, such as Amazons and African greys. Since cockatiels are so aerodynamic, owners must pay close attention to the condition of the bird's wing feathers and trim them regularly to keep the bird safe.

Once you've assembled your supplies, have your assistant drape the towel over his or her hand and catch your bird with the toweled hand. Grab the bird by the back of her head and neck, and wrap her in the towel. Have your assistant hold the sides of the bird's head securely with his or her thumb and index finger.

Enlist the help of an assistant to hold your bird while you do the trimming.

(Having the bird's head covered by the towel will calm her and will give her something to chew on while you clip her wings.)

Lay the bird on her back, being careful not to constrict or compress her chest (birds have no diaphragms to help them breathe, so their chests must be able to expand and contract) and spread her wing out carefully to look for blood feathers that are still grow-

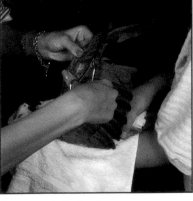

ing in. These can be identified by their waxy, tight look (new feathers in their feather sheaths resemble the end of a shoelace) and their dark centers or quills, which are caused by the blood supply to the new feather.

If your bird has a number of blood feathers, you may want to put off trimming her wings for a few days, because fully grown feathers cushion those just coming in from life's hard knocks. If your bird has only one or two blood feathers, leave a mature feather or two to protect the incoming blood feather and trim the rest accordingly. *Never trim a blood feather.*

To trim your bird's feathers, separate each one away from the other flight feathers and cut it individually (remember, the goal is to have a well-trimmed bird that's still able to glide down if she needs to). Use the primary coverts (the set of feathers above the primary flight feathers on your bird's wing) as a guideline as to how short you should trim.

To ensure your bird's safety, you must trim both wings. Cut the first six to eight flight feathers starting from the tip of the wing, and be sure to trim an equal number of feathers from each wing. Although some people think that a bird needs only one trimmed wing, this is incorrect and could actually cause harm to a bird that tries to fly with one trimmed and one untrimmed wing. Think of how off balance that would make you feel; your bird is no different.

If you do happen to cut or break a blood feather, remain calm. You must remove it and stop the bleeding, and panicking will do neither you nor your bird much good. You may want to pack the blood feather with styptic powder and take the bird to your veterinarian's office to have the blood feather removed.

To remove a blood feather, have your assistant hold the bird's wing steady. Then you need to take a pair of needle-nosed pliers and grasp the broken feather's shaft as close to the skin of your bird's wing as you can. With one steady motion, pull the feather out completely while your assistant applies equal and opposite pressure from the other side of the wing. After you've removed the feather, put a pinch of styptic powder on the feather follicle (the spot from which you pulled the feather) and apply direct pressure for a few minutes until the bleeding stops. If the bleeding doesn't stop after a few minutes of direct pressure, or if you can't remove the feather shaft, contact your avian veterinarian for further instructions.

Although it may seem like you're hurting your bird by removing the broken blood feather, consider this: A broken blood feather is like an open faucet. If the feather stays in, the faucet remains open and lets the blood out. Once removed, the bird's skin generally closes up behind the feather shaft and shuts off the faucet.

Now that you've successfully trimmed your bird's wing feathers, congratulate yourself. You've just taken a great step toward keeping your bird safe. But don't rest on your laurels just yet; you must remember to check your bird's wing feathers every month and retrim them periodically (about four times a year as a minimum).

Be particularly alert after a molt, because your bird will have a whole new crop of flight feathers that need attention. You'll be able to tell when your bird is due for a trim when she starts becoming bolder in her flying attempts. Right after a wing trim, a pet bird generally tries to fly and finds she's unsuccessful at the attempt. She will keep trying, though, and may surprise you one day with a fairly good glide across her cage or off her play gym. If this happens, get the scissors and trim those wings immediately. Otherwise, your beloved pet could fly away and never be seen again.

> **GROOMING TIPS**
>
> Groom your pet in a quiet, well-lit place.
>
> Have all the necessary grooming supplies close by before you begin.
>
> Make sure you have styptic powder on hand.
>
> Check wings and toenails regularly to see if they need retrimming.
>
> Consider having an avian veterinarian or other experienced person groom your bird.

Nail Trimming

While your assistant has the bird in the towel, trim the bird's nails. Some birds, such as lutino cockatiels, have

light-colored nails, which make it easier for owners to
see where the nail stops and the blood and nerve supply (or quick) begins. In lutinos, the quick is generally
seen as a pink color inside the nail. Owners of other
parrot species will have to pare down their birds' nails
carefully to ensure that they do not cut the quick.

*Trim your bird's
nails in the
smallest incre-
ments possible,
removing only
the hook on each
nail.*

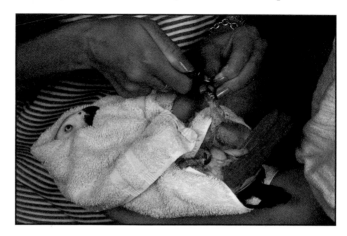

You will need to remove only tiny portions of the nail
to keep your pet's claws trimmed. Generally, a good
guideline to follow is to only remove the hook on each
nail, and to do this in the smallest increments possible.
Stop well before you reach the quick. If you do happen
to cut the nail short enough to make it bleed, apply
styptic powder, followed by direct pressure, to stop the
bleeding.

Bathing

Offer your bird a chance to bathe every day. This can
be accomplished in several ways. Pet stores sell baths
that attach to the side of a bird cage. If you own a kind of
bird that will get in this bath or is small enough to get
in, it's a good way to offer a bath because it keeps the
mess under control. Most small-to-medium-sized birds,
such as Finches, Canaries, Parrotlets, Cockatiels and
Quaker Parrots, will take a bath in a shallow dish. Make
sure the water just covers your bird's feet and that she
can easily get out of the bath dish. Birds cannot swim
and may have difficulty flying with wet feathers.

Most larger birds, and some small-to-medium-sized birds as well, enjoy bathing in the mist of a spray bottle. Always use fresh, warm water to spray your bird. Establish a routine and use the same spray bottle every time; use that bottle for nothing else to reduce the risk of exposing your bird to a dangerous chemical.

chapter 9

Your Avian
Veterinarian

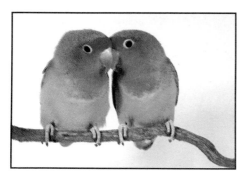

As a caring owner, you want your bird to have good care and the best chance at living a long, healthy life. To that end, you will need to locate a veterinarian who understands the special medical needs of birds with whom you can establish a good working relationship.

Selecting an Avian Veterinarian

Consider the following criteria when selecting an avian veterinarian.

- Does the hospital seem equipped to treat birds?
- Are the staff members pleasant, professional and knowledgeable?
- Do staff members own birds? Does the veterinarian?
- Is the veterinarian a member of the Association of Avian Veterinarians?

- Does the veterinarian seem competent and caring?

- Does he or she discuss your bird's case with you in terms that you can understand?

- Is the veterinarian open to answering questions from you?

- Are fees discussed openly and frankly?

- How does the hospital handle emergency cases?

It's important to establish a good relationship with an avian veterinarian before your bird needs emergency care. If the veterinarian knows your bird and already has his medical history, treatment will not be delayed. You should also be familiar with the location of the veterinarian's office and how to get there quickly. Additionally, you will feel more confident and less stressed if you and your veterinarian know each other.

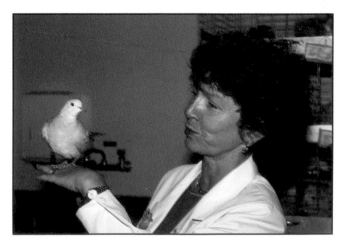

Locate a well-recommended avian veterinarian before you bring home a new pet bird.

You have to locate the best avian veterinarian for your bird before you can establish this important relationship. If you don't know an avian veterinarian in your area, ask the seller of your bird where he or she takes his or her birds. (Breeders and bird stores usually have avian veterinarians on whom they depend.) Talk to other bird owners you know and find out who they take their pets to, or call bird clubs in your area for referrals. The members can all give you their advice. Consider it all carefully and if more than one veterinarian has been recommended, interview each one yourself to form your own opinion.

If you don't belong to a bird club, check an annual issue of *Birds USA*, which you can find at most pet stores. In the back is a directory of avian veterinarians. You can also ask regular veterinarians in your area for a recommendation, or call a nearby zoo and ask to speak with the bird curator, who may be able to help. You can also check with regular veterinarians for the name and phone number of a bird rehabilitator in your area. This person will be another excellent source of information for an avian veterinarian.

If you don't have bird-owning friends or you can't locate a bird club, another good bet is the phone book. Read the advertisements for veterinarians carefully, and try to find one who specializes in birds. Many veterinarians who have an interest in treating birds will join the Association of Avian Veterinarians (AAV) and advertise themselves as members of this organization.

Once you've received your recommendations or found likely candidates in the telephone book, start calling the veterinary offices to make an appointment for your bird to have an evaluation. This visit will provide the veterinarian with a chance to see your bird under "normal" conditions. Your bird's medical history can be taken and filed for future reference, and the veterinarian can conduct some diagnostic tests (if appropriate) to gather additional information on your pet's health.

When you're calling to set up the appointment, ask the receptionist how many birds the doctor sees in a week

THE ASSOCIATION OF AVIAN VETERINARIANS

The Association of Avian Veterinarians (AAV) was founded in 1980 by a group of veterinarians who wanted to provide educational opportunities for veterinarians who worked with birds. Initially, 175 veterinarians from the United States and Canada joined the group, but the AAV now has more than 3,000 members in 43 countries around the world.

The AAV educates its members and the general public as to all aspects of avian medicine and surgery by offering conferences, practical labs, avicultural programs, client education brochures and a professional magazine devoted to all aspects of avian medicine. The AAV also provides funding for a variety of topics of interest to aviculture and avian medicine. Some veterinarians have taken and passed a special examination that entitles them to call themselves avian specialists.

or month, how much an office visit costs, and what payment options are available (cash, credit card, check or time payments).

If you like the answers you receive from the receptionist, make an appointment to have your bird evaluated. Make a list of any questions you want to ask the doctor regarding diet, how often your bird's wings and nails should be clipped or how often you should bring the bird in for an examination.

FIRST APPOINTMENT

Plan to arrive a little early for your first appointment because you will be asked to fill out a patient information form. This form will ask you for your bird's name, his age and sex, the length of time you have owned him, your name, address and telephone number. The form may also ask you to express your opinion on the amount of money you would spend on your pet in an emergency, because this can help the doctor know what kind of treatment to recommend in such instances.

Your bird will be given a complete physical examination during his first visit to the avian veterinarian.

During the initial examination, the veterinarian will probably take his or her first look at your bird while he is still in his cage or carrier. The doctor may talk to you and your bird for a few minutes to give the bird an opportunity to become accustomed to him or her, rather than simply reaching right in and grabbing your pet. While the veterinarian is talking to you, he or she will check the bird's posture and his ability to perch.

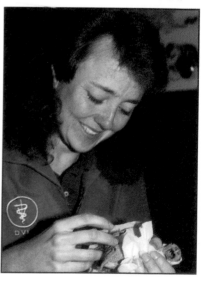

Next, the doctor should remove the bird from his carrier or cage and look him over carefully. He or she will give the bird a complete physical examination. The bird should be weighed, and the veterinarian will probably palpate (feel) your bird's body and wings for any lumps, bumps or deformities that require further investigation.

After the initial examination, you can discuss the questions you have about bird care with your avian veterinarian. You should also receive a recommendation for when to bring the bird back for his next examination. As you are leaving the hospital, you may want to make a follow-up appointment to have your bird's wings and nails trimmed to help protect him from accidental injury.

The Cost of Veterinary Care

One of the often overlooked aspects of bird ownership is the cost of veterinary care. Routine veterinary care for a pet bird may cost several hundred dollars a year, and emergency care to treat serious illnesses or injuries can cost even more.

When you take your bird in for emergency care, one of the questions you may be asked is how much you want to spend on care for your pet. It may also appear on the new patient form you fill out the first time you take your bird for a routine examination. Be honest when you answer this question because your answer can help the veterinarian and other hospital personnel assess and treat your pet. Know, too, that most veterinarians expect payment at the time services are rendered to your pet. If this will be a problem, tell the staff immediately so that alternate arrangements can be made as quickly as possible without delaying care for your pet.

How do you afford the cost of veterinary care for your pet bird? Some bird owners set up a special savings account or designate a certain credit card to be used only for veterinary expenses.

Your Bird's Health Care Team

In cases of accident or serious injury, you, your veterinarian and your veterinarian's staff will work together as your bird's health care team to give him the best chance to recover. In addition to working together during times of crisis, you need to help your veterinarian keep your bird in good health by observing him daily, feeding him a balanced diet, making sure he sees the veterinarian for regular checkups and ensuring that he is kept safe from accidents.

part three

Beyond the Basics

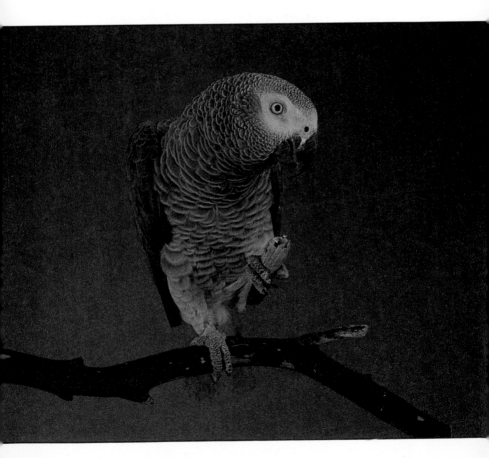

chapter 10

Resources

For more information on bird first aid and health care, look for these books at your local library, bookstore or pet store:

Books
ABOUT PET BIRD HEALTH

Doane, Bonnie Munro. *The Parrot in Health and Illness: An Owner's Guide.* New York: Howell Book House, 1991.

Gallerstein, Gary A. DVM. *Bird Owner's Home Health and Care Handbook.* New York: Howell Book House, 1984.

Gallerstein, Gary A. DVM. *The Complete Bird Owner's Handbook.* New York: Howell Book House, 1994.

Gerstenfeld, Sheldon L. VMD. *The Bird Care Book.* Reading, Mass.: Addison-Wesley Publishing Co., 1989.

Hawcroft, Tim BVSc, MACVSc, MRCVS. *First Aid for Birds.* New York: Howell Book House, 1994.

Randolph, Elizabeth. *The Basic Bird Book.* New York: Fawcett Crest Books, 1989.

About Toxic Plants

Alber, John I. and Delores M. *Baby-Safe Houseplants and Cut Flowers*. Highland, Ill.: Genus Books, 1990.

American Medical Association's Handbook of Poisonous and Injurious Plants. Chicago: American Medical Association, 1985.

Morelli, Jim. *Poison!* Kansas City: Andrews and McMeel, 1997.

Avian Veterinary Textbooks

Altman, Robert B. DVM; Susan L. Clubb DVM; Gerry M. Dorrestein DVM, PhD; and Katherine Quesenberry DVM. *Avian Medicine and Surgery*. Philadelphia: W.B. Saunders Co., 1997.

Ritchie, Branson W. DVM, PhD, Greg J. Harrison DVM, and Linda R. Harrison. *Avian Medicine: Principles and Application*. Lake Worth, Fla.: Wingers Publishing Inc., 1994.

Rosskopf, Walter J. Jr. DVM and Richard W. Woerpel MS, DVM. *Diseases of Cage and Aviary Birds*. Baltimore: Williams and Wilkens, 1996.

Magazines

Bird Talk
P.O. Box 57347
Boulder, CO 80322-7347

Bird Times
7-L Dundas Circle
Greensboro, NC 27499-0765

Birds USA
Look for it in your local bookstore or pet store.

Online Resources

Bird-specific sites have been cropping up regularly on the Internet. These sites offer pet bird owners the opportunity to share stories about their pets, along with trading helpful hints about bird care.

If you belong to an online service, look for the pet site (it may be included in more general topics, such as "Hobbies and Interests," or more specifically "Pets") If you have Internet access, ask your Web browser software to search for "pet bird health" or "parrot health."

Web Sites

These sites on the World Wide Web are just a few of those that may be of interest to bird owners who are concerned about their pets' health:

Alternative medicine:
http://www.altvetmed.com
This site is a good resource for owners who are seeking information on alternative, complimentary and holistic care for pets.

American Animal Hospital Association:
http://www.healthypet.com
This site offers pet care information and veterinary resources.

American Veterinary Medical Association:
http://www.avma.org
This site offers care information on a variety of companion animals, including pet birds.

Association of Avian Veterinarians:
http://www.aav.org
This site offers information on avian medicine and resources to help locate avian veterinarians in a particular area.

Bird Talk and *Bird Breeder* magazines:
http://www.petchannel.com/birds/default.asp
This site offers information on bird care and breeding from the publisher of *Bird Talk* magazine. *Bird Breeder*, a magazine aimed at the professional bird breeder, is available only online.

NetVet Veterinary Resources:
http://netvet.wustl.edu
This site offers a wide range of veterinary and animal-related resources.

Organizations

The following associations are interested in avian health and behavior.

American Animal Hospital Association
P.O. Box 150899
Denver, CO 80215-0899

American College of Veterinary Behaviorists
Dept. of Small Animal Medicine and Surgery
Texas A&M University
College Station, TX 77843-4474

American Veterinary Medical Association
1931 N. Meacham Rd., Suite 100
Schaumburg, IL 60173

Association of Avian Veterinarians
P.O. Box 811720
Boca Raton, FL 33481

Index